DRESS AND CARE

OF

THE FEET;

SHOWING

THEIR NATURAL SHAPE AND CONSTRUCTION; THEIR
USUAL DISTORTED CONDITION; HOW CORNS, BUNIONS,
FLAT FEET, AND OTHER DEFORMITIES ARE CAUSED,
WITH INSTRUCTIONS FOR THEIR PREVENTION
OR CURE.

ALSO,

DIRECTIONS FOR DRESSING THE FEET WITH COMFORT
AND ELEGANCE, AND MANY USEFUL HINTS TO
THOSE WHO WEAR, AS WELL AS THOSE WHO
MAKE FOOT-COVERINGS.

A History of Shoemaking

Shoemaking, at its simplest, is the process of making footwear. Whilst the art has now been largely superseded by mass-volume industrial production, for most of history, making shoes was an individual, artisanal affair. 'Shoemakers' or 'cordwainers' (cobblers being those who repair shoes) produce a range of footwear items, including shoes, boots, sandals, clogs and moccasins – from a vast array of materials.

When people started wearing shoes, there were only three main types: open sandals, covered sandals and clog-like footwear. The most basic foot protection, used since ancient times in the Mediterranean area, was the sandal, which consisted of a protective sole, attached to the foot with leather thongs. Similar footwear worn in the Far East was made from plaited grass or palm fronds. In climates that required a full foot covering, a single piece of untanned hide was laced with a thong, providing full protection for the foot, thus forming a complete covering. These were the main two types of footwear, produced all over the globe. The production of wooden shoes was mainly limited to medieval Europe however – made from a single piece of wood, roughly shaped to fit the foot.

A variant of this early European shoe was the clog, which were wooden soles to which a leather upper was attached. The sole and heel were generally made from one piece of maple or ash two inches thick, and a little longer and broader than the desired size of shoe. The outer side of the sole and heel was fashioned with a long chisel-edged implement, called the clogger's knife or stock; while a second implement, called the groover, made a groove around the side of the sole. With the use of a 'hollower', the inner sole's contours were adapted to the shape of the foot. In even colder climates, such designs were adapted with furs wrapped around the feet, and then sandals wrapped over them. The Romans used such footwear to great effect whilst fighting in Northern Europe, and the native Indians developed similar variants with their ubiquitous moccasin.

By the 1600s, leather shoes came in two main types. 'Turn shoes' consisted of one thin flexible sole, which was sewed to the upper while outside in and turned over when completed. This type was used for making slippers and similar shoes. The second type united the upper with an insole, which was subsequently attached to an out-sole with a raised heel. This was the main variety, and was used for most footwear, including standard shoes and riding boots.

Shoemaking became more commercialized in the mid-eighteenth century, as it expanded as a cottage industry. Large warehouses began to stock footwear made by many small manufacturers from the area. Until the nineteenth century, shoemaking was largely a traditional handicraft, but by the century's end, the process had been almost completely mechanized, with production occurring in large factories. Despite the obvious economic gains of mass-production, the factory system produced shoes without the individual differentiation that the traditional shoemaker was able to provide.

The first steps towards mechanisation were taken during the Napoleonic Wars by the English engineer, Marc Brunel. He developed machinery for the mass-production of boots for the soldiers of the British Army. In 1812 he devised a scheme for making nailed-boot-making machinery that automatically fastened soles to uppers by means of metallic pins or nails. With the support of the Duke of York, the shoes were manufactured, and, due to their strength, cheapness, and durability, were introduced for the use of the army. In the same year, the use of screws and staples was patented by Richard Woodman. However, when the war ended in 1815, manual labour became much cheaper again, and the demand for military equipment subsided. As a consequence, Brunel's system was no longer profitable and it soon ceased business.

Similar exigencies at the time of the Crimean War stimulated a renewed interest in methods of mechanization and mass-production, which proved longer lasting. A shoemaker in Leicester, Tomas Crick, patented the design for a riveting machine in 1853. He also introduced the use of steam-powered rolling-machines for hardening leather and cutting-machines, in the mid-1850s. Another important factor in shoemaking's mechanization, was the introduction of the sewing machine in 1846 – a development which revolutionised so many aspects of clothes, footwear and domestic production.

By the late 1850s, the industry was beginning to shift towards the modern factory, mainly in the US and areas of England. A shoe stitching machine was invented by the American Lyman Blake in 1856 and perfected by 1864.

Entering in to partnership with Gordon McKay, his device became known as the McKay stitching machine and was quickly adopted by manufacturers throughout New England. As bottlenecks opened up in the production line due to these innovations, more and more of the manufacturing stages, such as pegging and finishing, became automated. By the 1890s, the process of mechanisation was largely complete.

Traditional shoemakers still exist today, especially in poorer parts of the world, and do continue to create custom shoes. In more economically developed countries however, it is a dying craft. Despite this, the shoemaking profession makes a number of appearances in popular culture, such as in stories about shoemaker's elves (written by the Brothers Grimm in 1806), and the old proverb that 'the shoemaker's children go barefoot.' Chefs and cooks sometimes use the term 'shoemaker' as an insult to others who have prepared sub-standard food, possibly by overcooking, implying that the chef in question has made his or her food as tough as shoe leather or hard leather shoe soles. Similarly, reflecting the trade's humble beginnings, to 'cobble' can mean not only to make or mend shoes, but 'to put together clumsily; or, to bungle.'

As is evident from this short introduction, 'shoemaking' has a long and varied history, starting from a simple means of providing basic respite from the elements, to a fully mechanised and modern, global trade. It is able to provide a fascinating insight not only into fashion, but society, culture and climate more generally. We hope the reader enjoys this book.

PREFACE.

———◆———

THE object of this little treatise is to bring before the popular attention some ideas concerning the feet that are not generally familiar; to exhibit the producing causes of the common deformities and discomforts to which they are subject; to show the best means of preserving their natural shape and condition, or of restoring it as far as possible when lost; and to suggest better methods for their dress and general treatment, in order to their more perfect health, beauty, and performance of function.

The subject has already received some little attention. Some time about the beginning of the present cen-

tury Dr. Peter Camper, of Amsterdam—a distinguished
man of his time—wrote a short dissertation upon the
"Best Form of Shoe," which was eventually translated
and published in England in 1861, in connection with
a larger work by Mr. James Dowie. Dr. Camper's
essay was excellent as a first effort in this direction,
furnishing some ideas upon the form of the foot and
the defect of its covering, which still remain hardly
less just and appropriate. Mr. Dowie added some
good suggestions, and faithfully exposed the faults of
the foot-gear worn by the British army and the hum -
bler classes; but a considerable portion of his book
was taken up in the explanation and advocacy of
elasticated leather—an article of his own invention—
while the whole was written in a style too difficult to
be generally read.

Another work published in England was the " Book
of the Feet,", by J. Sparkes Hall, issued a few years
previous to that of Mr. Dowie. Though very interesting as a concise *history* of the shoemaking art, it

touched but slightly upon those abuses of the feet with which shoemaking is connected.

But a late essay directly upon the subject, by Prof. Hermann Meyer, of Zurich, Switzerland, has a value superior in this respect to that of all the preceding ones.

The present writer has intended to include all the important ideas of previous writers on the subject, together with such information as could be gathered from medical and other works, but going farther and adding such original notions as the observation and thought of his own mind could supply, with the purpose of making the whole as thorough and complete as possible, both from the point of view of the *physiologist* and that of the practical *shoemaker*.

The book is not written in the dignified style of a professor, nor with literary correctness; but it is hoped the ideas contained, and the nature of the subject-matter, will make it readable. It is addressed to those who desire comfort for their feet, and no less to those who wish to see them handsome in form and tastefully dressed.

As first prepared, the matter, under a different title, was printed in a trade journal—the *Shoe and Leather Reporter*—in 1868, since which a careful revision has improved and adapted it for its present form.

CONTENTS.

CHAPTER I.

DRESS AND CARE OF THE FEET.

THE human foot, it appears to us, is one of those members of the body that have never received their due share of consideration. Like certain *downtrodden* members of the *social* body, it seems to have been looked upon as having fewer "rights that were entitled to respect" than those organs which occupy a higher place, as the hands and eyes. No other part has been so abused by pinching, squeezing, chafing, freezing, and *corning*. The waist, of one sex especially, has suffered a good deal of compression, but not so much, we think as has the foot. It might perhaps be contended that the lowest parts of the system perform a function equally necessary with that of those above them and are therefore entitled to as tender care; but whether this be so or not, it is at least certain they are "pressed to earth" in a way that is wrong; and knowing this, it shall be our duty to set forth their wrongs and rights as well as we may, hoping to effect some improvement in the manner of their treatment.

The natural object and intention of the foot is the support of the body, and the carrying of it, in all its movements, lightly easily, safely and gracefully.   To this object it is as beautifully and wonderfully adapted as the eye and ear, those special objects of wonder, to the functions performed by them.   Its perfection may be most frequently seen in the graceful steps of the dance, though often also in the ordinary walk, while its capabilities may be judged of by the fact, not so generally known, that men deprived of their hands have succeeded in making their toes do the work of the fingers in writing.   Anatomy recognizes the fact, that in the number and character of the bones, joints, and muscles of the foot and leg, and the connection of the femur or thigh-bone at the pelvis, there is a strict similarity or correspondence with those of the hand and arm, and the connection of the latter at the shoulder-blade.   This justifies the conclusion, that all the variety of motion, and complete adaptation to an infinite number of uses, which exists in the hand, exists also to a less degree in the foot, and can be brought out and exhibited, much of it at least, under circumstances requiring its development.   There is no reason for scepticism as to the foot's concealed powers—none for withholding the admiration due to its perfect performance of the offices for which it is designed.

Nature, when allowed free scope for her work, does it

thoroughly and handsomely. Healthy children are born with arched insteps and straight toes. Notice the foot of the little urchin who runs barefoot in summer time around the outskirts of our cities and villages, and there is no fault to be found with it. Though the parents' feet have flat insteps, crooked toes, and big joints, those of the child are regular-shaped and sound. There seems to be an intention to give every one a fair start in the race of life with good pedal extremities. It is not at all probable that old father Adam went perambulating about his garden with the " hollow of his foot making a hole in the ground," or that his great toes pointed off in the direction of the little ones, as though they had a secret affinity for them, while the others were forced upward out of place, in order to cover up the affair ; nor that our beautiful mother Eve wandered among the flowers with *her* feet disfigured by corns and large joints. If they had been, would the serpent have cultivated her acquaintance in the way he did ? On the contrary, does not every painter and sculptor represent her with feet beautiful and shapely, like every other feature of her person ? Did the old Greek, Phidias, make flat feet on his statues, and ornament them with corns and callosities ? Did old Hércules have a big toe-joint on which to rest his club ? Or did the ancients of the Golden Age know about such things at all ? The Art of the world has never recognized them as beautiful or natural. We venture to say that in all the painting and sculpture of the past they cannot be found. They are entirely unnatural and deformed, belonging to the days of modern civilization. Nature makes her feet, except in rare instances, with arches well-marked and strong, and toes that point directly forward in the line of the foot's length. Yet the deformities spoken of are very common at the present time, and in this most intelligent part of the world. We believe, judging from a dozen years' experience in the making of boots and shoes for individual feet, that those more or less deformed constitute the rule, and the healthy and well-formed ones the exception. Such disfigurements and distortions are thrust upon our attention every day—crooked feet—short, stumpy feet—feet that tread inward, and those that tread only on the outside edge—flat feet—crippled feet—and feet so disproportioned that the part which should be an inch smaller than the instep is often half an inch larger—feet with large ankles, and feet with long heels—swelled feet, and feet that are nothing but bones—feet that turn inward and outward, and backward —feet with flat insteps—with big joints—with great toes that lie crosswise of the smaller ones—with small ones that grow over each other—with nails grown in, or to one side —with hard corns, and soft corns, little and big—with callosities on insteps, and heels, and ankles—with chilblains all over—feet with weak ankles that have lost their uprightness—sweaty feet—sensitive feet that take cold by wetting, and give their owner a consumption—and dirty feet that deserve to be diseased if they are not.

The causes of these depravities, diseases, and deformities are many and various. Thick and stiff leather coverings have had much to do with corns and callosities. False taste and fashions, bad habits of changing shoes, unnatural-shaped lasts, awkwardness in gait and movement, muscular weakness, and perhaps other causes that we do not yet know, have combined to produce flat insteps, crooked toes, large joints, weak ankles, and all the rest.

The subject is one in which all who have not lost their feet are more or less interested. To those who have children it is more especially important. While much may be done to reform the feet of adult persons, and it is intended to hold out all possible encouragement to them to attempt it, still it is with the children that the main work of correcting, improving, and educating must be effected. If a child's feet are trained up in the way they should *go*, they will not be likely, when they are older, to depart from it, and incur those penalties appropriately attached to an abuse of the foot's nature.

The particular causes of the more important of these troubles will be shown in the succeeding chapters, and suggestions for their remedy or prevention given.

CHAPTER II.

Natural Position of the Toes—Anatomical Argument—correspondence of Foot and Hand—Necessity of Freedom for the Toes—Criticism on Forms of Sole.

ONE of the worst of the distortions of the feet is the obliquity or bending of the great toe toward the outside, a fault with which several troublesome affections are often connected, besides the more prominent one, the enlargement of the joints.

To be convinced that this is a deformity, and of the *extent* to which it is so, let any one notice the shape and natural position of a child's foot, before it has been altered by forcing into a falsely-shaped shoe. *The toes will be found lying straight forward in the line of the foot's length,* with plenty of room for them to touch the ground without pressing against each other. This is plainly the case with every barefoot boy who is running about the streets or over the farm. There are no cramped toes ; on the contrary, they sometimes appear to be separated more than necessary, and the great toe, instead of inclining toward the outside of the foot, seems to be almost turning to the opposite direction.

All art, as already noticed in the first chapter, recognizes the right of the toes to sufficient space to touch the surface upon which they tread. It does not crowd them or turn them aside from their natural straightness.* An observation of the best specimens of statuary will confirm the assertion, *that the great toe ought, naturally, to lie pointing directly forward, in such a position that a line drawn from the inner surface of the heel past the ball or joint will be nearly parallel to it.* It would seem that such a statement is so nearly self-evident that every one must instantly admit its truth, and ought to be aware of it without argument. Yet we doubt that it is commonly recognized, or that the mass of people ever really think of it. Nor do we suppose those who have thought of it have considered the matter to be of any importance, unless they happened to be afflicted with some of the troubles that accompany toe-distortion ; nor often then with any idea of removing or preventing those evils. It is certain that the shoe manufacturer and the last-maker have not had such a supposition clearly in mind, at least with any idea of changing the shape of the last accordingly. One manu-

* It is also true that many artists have been led to a mistake by observation of the adult foot, which has been more or less deformed by its coverings. In many works of art there is a larger joint than natural, and the great toe is turned aside sufficiently to bring all the toes close together, though not enough to be a positive distortion.

facturer who had been engaged in making boots and shoes for the feet of his customers during twenty years recently stated that, having drawings of thousands of feet, and always finding the big toe turned toward the outside, more or less, he never thought of it as being other than the foot's normal shape. This shows how common the deformity, as well as how uncommon the thought of what is the foot's true form according to nature.

A pamphlet called " *Why the Shoe Pinches,*" discussing this subject quite clearly, and with the authority of science, was written by Herrman Meyer, M.D., Professor of Anatomy in the University of Zurich. To it we are indebted for many of the most important ideas here contained, and for a presentation of the matter which first drew our earnest attention. It gives an anatomical argument, illustrated by diagrams, to show the proper form of the toes and forward part of the foot, which we will try to present in our own way.

The *metatarsal* bones are five of the longest bones of the foot, lying below, or in front of, what is commonly known as the instep, and filling the space between the instep and the toes, though, strictly speaking, they form a part of the whole instep. They are nearly parallel with each other, and to their forward ends the bones of the toes are attached, forming the back toe-joints, at the part called the bend of the foot. Where the great toe joins its metatarsal bone, is called the *ball* or *inside ball;* or, more strictly, it is the under surface which is so called. These metatarsal bones being straight, and so nearly parallel to· each other, it is a natural inference that the toe-bones attached to them should lie straight in front of them, on the same lines, and nearly parallel to each other also. In short, *they must do so*, in order that when covered with flesh they shall have room to touch the ground, or bend, without interfering. This would bring all the toes, and their meta-tarsal bones, parallel or nearly so, with a line drawn past the whole inside of the foot. They would thus be allowed space to grow naturally, to lie side by side, and perform

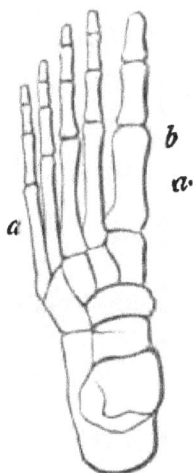

FIG. 1.—*a a*, METATARSAL BONES ; *b*, JOINT.

their proper functions without crowding or chafing, or inclining sideways in either direction. The diagram of a skeleton foot (copied from Professor Meyer's pamphlet) will show this more plainly than words.

It is claimed by the Professor, in this little book, that a line drawn from the middle of the heel—on the sole—under the centre of the ball or joint, should pass under the middle of the great toe, through its whole length. His reasoning for this idea is thus given :

" The great toe plays by far the most important part in walking, because when the foot is raised from the ground, with the intention of throwing it forward, we first raise the heel, then rest for a second on the great toe, and in lifting this from the ground the point of it receives a pressure which impels the body forward. Thus, in raising the foot, the whole of the sole is gradually, as it were, '*unrolled*,' up to the point of the great toe, which again receives an impetus by contact with the ground. The great toe ought, therefore, to have such a position as will admit of its being *unrolled* in the manner described ; that is to say, it must so lie that *the line of its axis, when carried backward, will emerge at the centre of the heel ;* and this is its position in the healthy foot."

The great toe certainly plays an important part in walking, and is therefore entitled to all necessary freedom. The position taken may be further strengthened by bringing forward the fact that all natural feet are slightly wider at the ball than at the instep, an inch and a half farther back ; that is, wider at the forward than at the back or upward ends of the metatarsal bones. This is readily seen

in the cut of a healthy foot, Fig. 2, and still more plainly
in that of the foot-skeleton, Fig. 3.

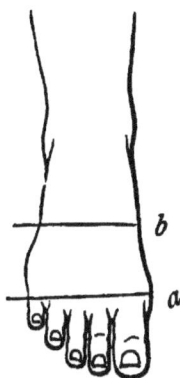

FIG. 2.

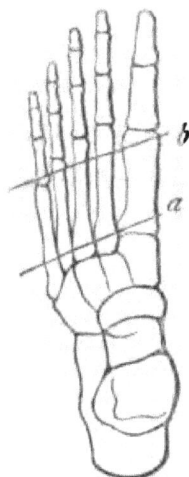

FIG. 3.

In each of these figures the difference in the width at
the points *a* and *b* is what we wish to be noticed. It is
argued above, with good reason, that the bone of the great
toe should lie directly forward of its metatarsal bone, on
the same line, which line, when carried back, passes under
the centre of the heel. And it is equally fair to infer that
the *smaller* toes should lie directly forward of *their* metatarsal bones, on the same lines. This would allow all the
toes to be spread a very little, as is apparent in Fig. 2, and
as the bones are spread in Fig. 3. There is thus a slight,
but distinct, gradual widening of the foot, from the middle
region to the ends of the toes, an idea which will be confirmed in every child's foot that may be observed.

The correspondence between the bones of the foot and leg and those of the hand and arm also give countenance to this notion. The *metacarpal* bones of the hand are those which answer to the *metatarsal* bones of the foot ; and that they are wider apart at their forward ends than at their base or origin, is observable from the skeleton hand Fig. 4, and from the hand having the thumb turned under, Fig. 5.

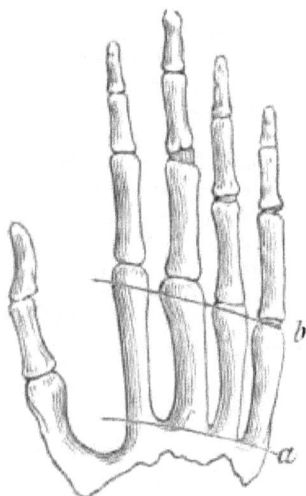

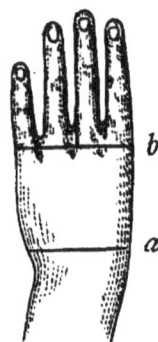

FIG. 4.   FIG. 5.

In this case, as in that of the foot, if the fingers lie directly forward of their metacarpal bones, they are slightly spread or separated. And the next fact to which attention is requested is, that we never think of forcing them into one position, or of confining them there, as is done with the toes—a treatment that would quickly destroy their usefulness, if attempted. They are allowed perfect freedom to close or separate ; to be pushed over to one side or the other, as occasion requires ; and to assume any natural position when unoccupied.

Now, although there is a greater demand for the liberty of the fingers, on account of the innumerable uses to which they are capable of being put, the difference between them and the toes, in this respect, is only a difference of degree ; and it is evident that *something*, more or less, of the same bad effect which would attend the cramping of the former, must, as it does, attend the confinement and squeezing undergone by the latter. It seems clear that in a state of nature the toes are left equally free to " spread themselves," or draw together when necessary, or to return to their proper places in line with the metatarsal bones, when there is nothing to draw them on one-side. In circumstances where they would not be interfered with, the large one would doubtless have the position given it by Professor Meyer, or, at least one very nearly the same ; that is, the line of the toes carried backward would touch the middle of the heel, and the whole inside of the foot would have a general appearance of straightness. This, it is repeated, is the form of the normal adult foot, and of the child's foot universally.

The only form of shoe which is absolutely correct, then, is one allowing this amount of freedom to the toes—not alone to the great one, but to all. The form recommended by Dr. Meyer, which is represented in Fig. 6, like every other now made distorts the little toe, compelling it to turn under toward the middle of the foot, and giving it that peculiar twist that almost every one may notice in his own.

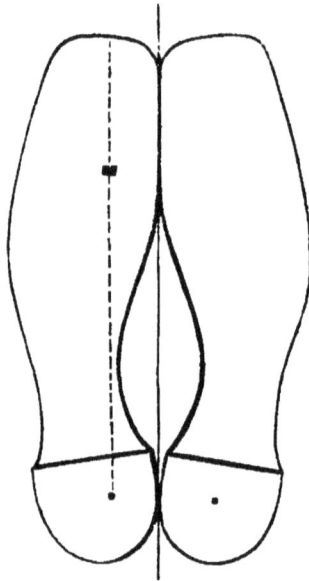

FIG. 6.—SHAPE OF SOLE GIVEN IN "WHY THE SHOE PINCHES."

This, however, is only a slight fault compared to the bending aside of the large toe, and is mentioned mainly to show that neither that form nor any other gives to *all* the toes the freedom which properly belongs to them. The true standard form is one that will not compel *any* of them to be cramped or bent aside, nor press injuriously upon any part of the foot; and to this form it should be the shoemaker's endeavour to approximate as nearly as possible.

But such a shape as would fulfil this requirement has never been realised since the days of the ancient sandal And the problem for the shoemaker to solve is to create a covering that will give the freedom and ease of the old sandal, combined with neatness and elegance of fit, with protection from dirt, cold, and dampness ; and with propriety and beauty throughout. It will be something considerably different from any now worn, and may tax his ingenuity to a greater extent than is supposed. Professor Meyer is right concerning the form of its sole at the *inside ;* but the curve at the outside is too much like the common style to be exactly the right thing. There seems to be required a more abrupt curve at a point somewhat farther forward than where the widest part is usually found

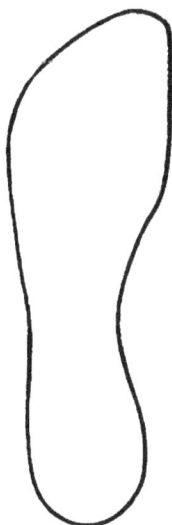

FIG. 7.

—a curve approaching more nearly to an obtuse angle, something like what is represented in Fig. 7.

Thus, modifying, or adding to, the form of sole given by Dr. Meyer, we present it as the most perfect one we are now able to suggest, and one the correctness of which is confirmed by all the facts of anatomy, and by everything bearing upon the subject.

As to what is theoretically right, then, we not only indorse all that is urged by the author quoted, but go farther, and claim for little toes, as well as great ones, the right to grow as straight as nature intended them, and to spread as freely as circumstances may require. There is a point, however—one of practice, not theory—upon which we may perhaps be said to partially disagree, and which will be explained farther on. It is designed now to show some of the bad results of a failure to conform the shape of the boot or shoe to that of the foot ; and afterward to consider what can be done in the way of improvement.

CHAPTER III.

Distortion of the Toes and Joint—Various Causes—Want of Harmony between Shape of Foot and Shape of Shoe—Grown-in Nails —Influence of Stockings, Narrow-Toed Soles, High Heels, and Changing of Shoes—Faults of Lasts.

THE doctrine concerning the shape and position of the toes is considered to be made sufficiently clear by what has been already advanced. As the best illustration of it, we copy from Dr. Meyer's book a cut of the natural, healthy foot of a child (Fig. 8), in which the line of the great toe, continued backward, passes under the middle of the heel. By the side of this is placed a shoe-sole of the common form (Fig. 9), and which plainly does not harmonize with the shape of the foot. From the ball forward instead of being straight on the inside line, it slants off obliquely toward the middle of the toe, making as great an inclination or curve on that side as on the outside. As the toes of the foot cannot force the upper of a boot over the sole to any great extent, the form of the sole determines the shape in which the toes shall lie when they are inside the boot. The line $c\ d$, in the diagram, shows where the great toe ought to be ; but, far from being there, it is turned aside into the line *c e*, a position entirely unnatural. We will here quote again from the book, taking the liberty to italicize :

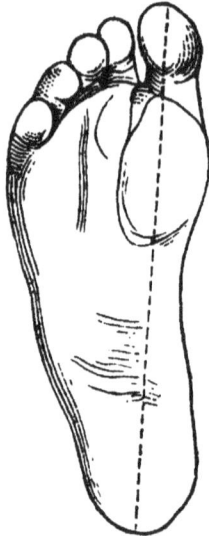

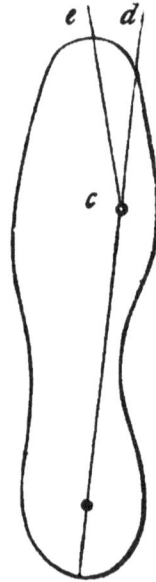

FIG. 8.   FIG. 9

" It is quite clear that the foot must get into the shoe ; and if the shoe differs in shape from the foot, it is no less plain that the foot, being the more pliable, must necessarily adapt itself to the shape of the shoe. If, then, fashion prescribes an *arbitrary* form of shoe, she goes far beyond her province, and in reality arrogates to herself the right of determining the shape of the foot.

" But the foot is a part of the body, and must not be

changed by fashion; for our body is a gift, and its several parts are beautifully adapted to the purposes for which they were intended.

" If, therefore, we in any way change its normal form, *not only do we not improve, but we actually disfigure it.*

" We do not, indeed at first sight, perceive the arrogant absurdity of which fashion is guilty in going so far as to determine the shape of our feet, because we are not alive to the fact that the case is *peculiar* to the feet. We only see it influencing the shape of the shoe, and come to the conclusion that it may regulate this, as well as the cut of the coat. To this prevalent opinion we yield, regardless of the influence on the shape of the shoe, and thereby on the foot. As well, indeed, might fashion one day come to the conclusion that *fingers* are inelegant, and decree that henceforth the hand be squeezed into a conical leather bag; as well, indeed, might she in one of her freaks, forbid the display of our arms, and bind them firmly to our bodies, like those of children in swaddling clothes.

" The shoe ought to *protect* the foot, but it has no right to *distort its shape.*"

Seeing, therefore, that the common form of boots and shoes, as now made, is not the true one, and that it arbitrarily forces the great toe into a false position, it follows that all the bad effects resulting from this false position are to be attributed directly to the incorrect form of the last and shoe. The first of these is a crowding together

2—2

of all the toes, in which some are obliged to find their places *under*, and some *above*, the more ambitious of them sometimes pushing their nails through the upper leather, the rubbing and chafing they meet making them sore, while the more humble are glad to curl themselves down in any way that will give them a place of comfort.   When the crowding is not so great as to force them out of place there is still a constant pressure against each other that is liable to create corns between them.

Another effect is the *growing in*, or to *one side*, of the nails.   The boot-upper presses the flesh against the nail of the great toe on one side, while there is a similar pressure from the smaller toes on the opposite side, and between both, the nail is almost compelled to grow into the flesh, if it grows at all.   If the great toe gets the advantage, then the one next to it is likely to suffer in the same way, and all of them are liable to the same trouble.   When the nail grows so far that its edge turns downward, the pressure against the sole, in walking or standing, is a more aggravated discomfort.   Dr. Meyer says that " by degrees it [the toe] gets into a state of chronic inflammation, and may eventually become ulcerated, producing what is popularly known as 'proud flesh.'   The ailment not only interferes with the use of the foot, but too often requires, for its relief, medical, and even operative interference."   A surgical operation of this kind, which consists in removing the nail entirely, we are assured, by those who have seen it, is an intensely painful thing to witness, and cannot be less so to

be borne. The following description of the nature of the
trouble, and of the mode of treatment, is copied from Dr.
R. T. Trall, for the benefit of those who may wish to treat
it for themselves.

" *Onyxis.*—This distressing affliction consists in an in-
curvation of the toe-nail from a bruise or the pressure of a
tight shoe, producing inflammation and ulceration, and
followed eventually by fungous growths, or proud flesh,
which is excedingly tender and painful. The cure is slow
but certain. The foot must be frequently soaked in warm
water, until the soreness is so far abated that it can be
handled without pain ; then, with a probe, press pledgets
of lint as firmly as can be borne under the most detached
point of the nail, pressing them also between the nail and
projecting portions of the flesh, as far as possible. Cover
these with the wet compress, and apply a moderately tight
bandage over the whole, frequently wetting the whole with
warm, tepid, or cold water, as either temperature is most
agreeable. The lints are to be pressed farther and farther
under the nail, from time to time, and the foot should be
soaked and dressed once or twice daily. When portions
of the nail become free they may be cut off, and mild
caustics may be employed to remove fungous or indurated
growths, which do not yield to the other measures of
treatment."

A *slim*-toed shoe—one that is *thin,* and scant in the
upper—whatever be its width or shape, has a bad influence
upon the nails, not only by inciting them to grow in, but

by turning them down at the ends, and keeping them
constantly irritated and sore, a condition which effectually
prevents the toes from being of any use. The seller of
such an article will sometimes try to persuade the wearer
that it is a " good fit" when snug at the forward part,
however loose elsewhere ; and many persons are quite
willing to be persuaded in this way. But if they are wise
they will not attempt to wear anything that is not perfectly
easy to the toes, for these may be allowed all necessary
room, and still, if the fit is " just right," there will be no
wrinkling, nor any other bad appearance.

The next and most important of the difficulties springing from this source is the enlargement of the great-toe
joint. We continue to quote from Meyer :

" Not less important are the evils arising at the root of
the great toe from the same cause. It has already been
stated that the pressure of the upper leather pushes the
point of the great toe against the smaller toes. The joint
at the metatarsal bone thus becomes *bent aside,* so that it
forms a protuberance on the inner side of the foot. If the
point of the toe is now pressed against the ground in walking, this protuberance must be made still greater, and so
pressed more forcibly against the upper leather. At the
same time, moreover, the great transverse wrinkle in the
upper leather—the result of the bending of the toes—
presses directly on the same point, and the protuberance
at the root of the toe is thus constantly subjected to a two-
fold and very injurious pressure. In these circumstances

it is by no means wonderful that this joint becomes subject to a continual inflammation, which by extending to the bones must, in this situation, produce permanent and painful swellings, which become, in their turn, and even from slight causes, the source of inflammations and new growths of bone.

"In this manner arise those unseemly and painful swellings at the root of the great toe, which, either from mistaking their true nature, or from wilful deception, are called 'chilblains,' or 'gout,' just as one or the other term appears the most interesting. In many cases, moreover, this kind of inflammation of the bones, and their investing membrane, may lead to the formation of matter, *and eventually to the disease known as 'caries,' or ulceration of the bone.*"

Narrow-toed shoes furnish another influence strongly operating to produce large joints. The great toe is drawn farther than usual toward the others, and its joint thrown out in the opposite direction. All the toes are more crowded, until some of them are forced out of place while corns and grown-in nails are developed or made worse. Width at the ball alone will not prevent these effects. French and English styles are in this respect often pernicious. The whole tendency of narrow toes is toward deformity ; and those who cannot because they happen to be the style, refuse to wear them, should make up their minds to accept the consequences with a good grace.

Another great cause of the prominence and swelling of the joint—which our author alludes to, but gives it hardly any of its real importance—is the backward pressure of the toe by shoes that are too *short.* This, in addition to causing sore nails, crowds the toes still more closely together, and pushes the joint still farther inward, away from its proper place. To illustrate.

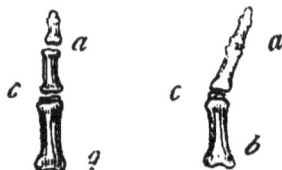

FIG. 10.   FIG. 11.

a, PHALANGES, OR BONES OF THE TOE; *b*, METATARSAL BONE; *c*, JOINT.

Supposing these to represent the bones of the great toe and its metatarsal bone—which, in their normal position, are on the same line—we can see that if the toe bones *a* are bent toward the other toes first, and then pushed backward, it necessarily forces out the joint in the only direction in which it *can* bend, which is inward. The greater and more constant the pressure against the end of the toe by the short boot or shoe, the larger the joint, and the more it will project from the inside of the foot; the more liable also to soreness, swelling, corns, bunions, inflammation, and settled disease, and the more awkward, ill-shaped, and uncomfortable, not only to walk with but to look upon.

High heels also do their share toward bringing on this deformity. They cause the foot to pitch downward on the toes, sometimes pushing it a size farther forward into the boot than it would go if the heel was only moderately high, thus creating the necessity for a *longer* boot. *The crowding of the toes is increased; and as they meet with resistance or a backward pressure from both sides and the end of the shoe*, at the same time that there is a *forward pressure from the heel* by the weight of the body, *of course the angle formed at the joint must be pushed out more acute, the foot* making room for itself by stretching and treading over the upper at the sides.

There is a peculiarity about the *Plumer* last recommending it in this particular. The heel, on the bottom, is quite convex, which allows the heel of the foot to settle down into that of the boot more than usual, and thus what appears to be a high heel, outside, feels, on the foot, to be no higher than one made upon ordinary lasts an eighth of an inch lower. There is hence so much less pressure upon the ends of the toes.

A false habit, tending in the same direction, is that of *changing* the shoes of children to make them wear evenly or prevent their treading over to one side at the heel. It is a practice productive of far more harm than good—a saving of shoe-leather at the foot's expense. *After one foot has shaped a shoe to itself, to put the other into it*

forcing the great toe into the curve made by the little toe *
and outside of the foot, must do much toward bending the
toe permanently out of place.   It should never be allowed
or proposed. Give children *right and left* shoes, and guard
against their wearing on one side by good firm counters·
It is their right, when obtainable, and anything less is
injustice.

While the foot is growing, it easily adapts itself to its
surroundings ; and by wearing short boots and shoes it
may be encouraged to grow into a bad shape in a few years.
Most old people have joints deformed in this way.   We
have also seen them on the feet of young and beautiful
women, where they seemed most sadly out of place. Young
feet are often forced to grow into uncomely shape through
the good intentions of parents, whose falsely-taught in-
stinct of beauty induces them to put as small a shoe on
the child's foot as it will bear, fearing that if left to itself
it will grow too long, or too wide, to be elegant in form.
The motive of this action is most commendable, but its
wisdom extremely doubtful and weak. Beauty, taste, elegance, are to be sought for everywhere and always. We
have not the least sympathy with any attempt to depreciate
them.   But they are not to be sought by counteracting
nature. On the contrary, nature is most trustworthy. If
not interfered with, she will make the foot grow in due proportion to the size of the whole body ; and every part will
be developed in the right proportion to itself.

" Children of a larger growth" continue to carry out the

same false idea by wearing as short and narrow a boot as they can squeeze their foot into with any degree of comfort. While the object is to obtain a handsome foot, *all such cramping inevitably defeats its purpose. The effect which it invaribly has and must have, is to make the joints project, and add from one-fourth to three-fourths of an inch to the foot's width,* leaving out of account the torture accompanying the process. Nobody will claim that large joints and extra width at this point make a good-looking foot, but they are the sure results, in greater or less degree according to the severity of the pinching, and the length of the time it is continued.

It is well to ascertain if *stockings* do not have some effect in giving a bad shape to this part of the foot, although made of such yielding materials that they may at first thought, appear harmless. Mr. James Dowie, in a work published in England some years since, speaking of the toes being cramped, crowded, bent, and piled over each other, attributes part of this result to the stocking, and recommends the wearing of one having *toes* on it—similar to the fingers on a glove. There is no reason to doubt that this conclusion is correct, for while a stocking that is loose may be drawn into almost any shape to suit the toes, one which is *tight, short, and narrow-toed, must, and does, draw the toes together and keep them so,* however favourable may be the form of the boot outside. It is a fact, too, that stockings are narrow and pointed at the toe ; almost universally. The suggestion of putting *toes* to them

is a good one.   But if this is thought to be taking too
much pains with such an article—though it is evidently
impossible to take too much pains in dressing any part of the
body so as to protect it from being injured in any manner
—it is perfectly easy to make the stocking *wider* at this
part, leaving it *nearly square, or with only a slight round-
ness at the end.*   This would be a very decided improvement, and cannot be urged too strongly.*

Like the defects of the shoe, those of the stocking must
be felt more seriously by children.   They are ignorant of
the matter, and would be careless and inattentive even if
they were not.   But if parents will half do their duty by
them, there is no reason why they should not grow up
with well-formed feet, thankful for the care which has saved
them from distortion and blessed them with pedal come-
liness.

There is here, also, a question of the comparative taste
and elegance of wide and narrow soles, which needs a
little discussion.   It is the practice with many persons to
wear as narrow a boot or shoe as they can, thinking we
suppose, that if they have not a narrow foot, they *ought
to have*, and that by putting it into a narrow boot they
prevent it from spreading.   As such a boot is and will be
*narrow at the toe, the effect is just the opposite of that in-
tended* as in the case of *short* ones.   *The toes are drawn
together, and the ball pushed out wider than before.*   Then
besides this tendency to *make* it wider, the foot *looks*

---

* We have lately seen stockings for sale that were nearly square-
toed, and these should obtain the preference in buying.

wider in a shoe that is too narrow for it, because it treads the upper over, and the narrow toe makes it appear all the wider by contrast. A *foot* that is narrow may wear a narrow-soled shoe with propriety; for a *wide* one to attempt to do so is foolish. We have seen a lady's boot trodden over so far that a hole had been worn through the upper on each side of the sole by its contact with the ground. The wearer doubtless thought it was necessary for her to wear a narrow sole to prevent her foot from spreading, and keep it in an elegant shape. She did not know that she was taking the most direct way to defeat her object, and that her true policy would have been to wear the widest-soled shoe she could get. This case was extreme, but it is quite common to see the upper worn through on *one* side from the same cause. The right kind of shoe for a wide foot is one so wide on the sole that the upper will project over it on the sides but slightly, and *with as great a width of the toe, in proportion to the ball, as there would be in a narrow one. Such a shoe will make the foot appear narrower, by contrast, than it really is*, and the greater the width of the toe, the more this effect is produced. Besides, the shoe or boot *keeps its proper shape* much better and longer when not too narrow or too short. If the *foot* be *short* proportionately, as well as wide, the covering should be of good *length*—at least a full size to spare at the toe, after being worn a few days and fitted, or broken in. These doctrines may not be readily accepted, but let any one who doubts give them a trial, and we are willing to be judged by the opinion formed afterward.

There are those who appear to urge the idea that broad soles are eminently proper always, and for everybody, which doctrine we do not endorse ; but we mean to say that persons who have wide feet naturally, or who have made them wide at the joints in the ways here pointed out, ought to wear wide soles. It is also quite certain that if people wore soles of the correct shape from childhood there would be a far less number than now of those feet, that require this extra width of sole, for nine-tenths of them *are forced into a width which they would not have by nature*, and, when once deformed, no pains taken in fitting them can make them look *well*, or like those which keep their proper shape.

A *narrow* foot must not be confounded with a *slim* one. Feet that are slim—that measure less than an average in circumference—are often found *wider* than most of those of the same length which are of medium size or fulness. These are feet that *spread*, and may generally be found on individuals of spare or muscular temperament. Such persons ought to wear boots made on wide lasts, with wide toes, though at the same time sufficiently slim to fit. As such lasts cannot easily be found ready-made, those having feet of this shape ought to possess a pair made expressly for themselves.

There is an opposite style of feet, those which are long and narrow, while they may be also *full*, or thick, verti-

cally. These are usually found on persons who are tall,
yet round, and fleshy in physique. They can wear boots
made on lasts that are comparatively narrow, such as may
be found at any shoe-shop. It is not intended to argue in
favour of any *unnecessary* width in either case, but simply
to urge the necessity, not only for comfort, *but especially
for elegance also*, of having sufficient width to accommodate the foot easily, aud preserve the natural shape of
both the foot and its covering.

Bad fashions of *lasts* have had much to do in producing
a deformed condition of the feet, as well as the false ideas
and tastes of the people. Shoemakers, and more especially
last-makers, who should have studied the nature of the
foot, and given the people, who looked to them for a correctly-shaped last and shoe, something truly and naturally
adapted to its purpose, have failed in this part of their
duty. The latter have made lasts of all varieties of shape
except the true one, while the maker of the shoe has made
a bad matter worse with his high and short heels.

Formerly the great majority of ladies' shoes and gaiters
were made upon lasts that were *straight*, and the same is
true even yet. Almost the whole of the cheaper kinds of
work got up in the manufactories is of this style. Slippers
are hardly ever seen made upon other than straight lasts.
The whole custom is a wrong one, for this reason ; the
middle of the toe of shoes made upon straight lasts is
nearer to the outside than it is in those made on rights-
and-lefts. Hence they draw the great toe farther toward

the outside of the foot than do those of the latter kind, *and have a greater effect in producing all the evils that go with deformed toes and joints.* No woman ought to be asked to wear them, nor should she allow herself to do so if those of another form can be obtained. Girls whose feet are growing cannot have them forced into straight shoes, especially if tight, without perpetrating a kind of tyranny very similar in character to that of the Chinese. Right-and-left boots and shoes are the natural right of all men, women, and children. Men and boys have, in this respect, the advantage over their sisters, as their foot apparel is almost wholly of the better shape. There is no reason why women and girls should not have the benefit of the improvement in form, though it is only a slight one, and they are counselled to take it whenever they can. In fact, there is no excuse for straight shoes, except that they can be made a little more cheaply—that is, there is a little less expense for the lasts used. They do not wear more evenly than the others—on the contrary, they are quite as liable, if not more so, to tread over at the heel. They never fit the foot so well in the hollow, at the instep, or on the side. There is no *necessity* for their existence, for there is no form of foot-covering but might be made on crooked lasts with equal facility. Ladies' slippers are believed to be the only article that is *always* made straight, and for these, right-and-left lasts, properly adapted to the purpose, might be used without the least difficulty. Considering these facts, and that there is but a slight advantage to the manufacturer, and to him only, in their production, and that the children and poorer class of women, who wear them the most helpless classes in the community—are almost compelled to deform their feet in doing so, it becomes a disgrace to the shoemaking profession that straight shoes are not abolished.

Many right-and-left lasts are made *so nearly straight* that the difference in form, and the benefit arising from it, amount to but very little. This must be remedied by the people learning what is to be desired, and making a demand for it. It is sometimes argued that the straighter the last is, the less liable is the foot to tread the boot over to one side ; but this we hold to be a fallacy, and that the liability to tread over, is determined by the shape of that part of the last between the heel and instep. The form of the *toe or forward part* has nothing to do with the matter. It is generally, however, an advantage to the foot, though not to the boot, if it succeeds in treading the latter over to the *outside.* It thus gives the boot a more distinctly right-and-left shape, and can hence more easily preserve its own. When it goes over *inside*, there is a good prospect of a big joint being soon produced.

The last-makers have given us toes of many styles, from the turn-up toes an inch longer than necessary, to the stub-toes half an inch shorter than the foot ; and from the round toe narrowed to a point, to the square one nearly or quite as wide as the ball. All that needs to be said of them is, that the wider they are, except the extreme just

3

noted, the better for the foot, at least while the present lasts are in use, and generally the handsomer also ; that the long toe is unnecessary, and therefore unhandsome ; while the short or stub toe is decidedly awkward and clumsy-looking, besides being injurious to the foot, and utterly unworthy of toleration by any person of sense or taste. The true and most tasteful shape will be found near the half-way point between the two extremes in each direction. Whether round or square is of no material consequence.

Here, then, we have found several causes for the deformities of the forward part of the foot—the crooked great toe, the cramped and distorted smaller ones, the corns between, the grown-in nails, the big joint, and the increased width. The cause first operating to produce them is the wrong shape of the shoe at the inside, which gives the oblique position to the great toe. Narrowness and shortness are stronger influences acting in the same direction, aided still further by extreme height of heels, by changing, by narrow-toed stockings, etc. And it is especially worthy of being noticed that the short and narrow toes, and the high heels often adopted to improve the foot's appearance, do thus inevitably defeat that purpose.

The attention of those who regard their own foot-comfort is earnestly directed to the points and reasoning presented in this chapter. Just as earnestly it is desired that those whose principal aim in dressing the foot is its beauty, elegance, and perfection of form, should give a thorough consideration to what has been said. Both classes will easily see that, in order to gain the object sought, there must be a reform in the shape and style of the foot's covering. The nature of that improvement is already partially shown—that is, as far as the toes are concerned —and will be shown fully in what is to follow.'

The cuts below, showing some of the worst deformities of the forward part of the foot, and adding the force of illustration to what has been said, are an appropriate con- clusion to this chapter. It will do no harm to contrast them with Fig. 8 and Fig. 3, previously given.

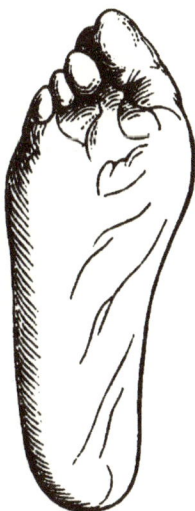

FIG. 12.

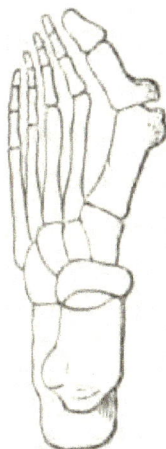

FIG. 13.

CHAPTER IV.

Prevention of Deformed Toes and Joint—New Forms of Sole—
Eureka Last—True Standard of Taste—How Distorted Great
Toe may be Straightened—Ancient and Medieval Foot-apparel—
Suggestions.

L ET us next endeavour to ascertain what shall be done
toward substituting an improved form of covering
for the present false style, as a method of *preventing* distortion of the toes and the evils connected with it; and
also inquire how far these deformities can be relieved by
proper effort after they have been induced.

The shape of sole previously described and illustrated
(Fig. 7) is taken to be as near the absolutely correct one
as anything that can now be devised, and to be approxi-
mated and realized as soon in the future as possible. It
is true that people should be capable of recognizing its
correctness, and of adopting it practically, at once; and,
doubtless, there are some who can conscientiously disre-
gard the strong tendency to conformity with the prevailing
false styles, and wear a boot or shoe which represents the

right idea, or one as near to it as it is possible for them to obtain. All such are earnestly advised to take this course, and continue it, both for their own good, and as a means of developing a sentiment in favour of the change.

But there are other people, in larger numbers, who will not be persuaded to attempt so much of a change without some encouragement from popular sympathy. These must not only be taught to know what is right and wrong in the matter, but be led to adopt the right through gradually approximating steps, that do not vary so far from the style at any time prevalent as to be unpleasantly *odd.* The eye must become accustomed to different forms, and first to those that deviate least from the present fashion. Bearing this in mind, what is the best improvement that can be made generally acceptable?

Our principal care is the preservation of the shape of the great toe and inside joint, not forgetting that the little toe is also entitled to care ; still, the great one is much the most important, and if only one can be properly attended to, the little one must wait its opportunity. Its deformity consists in being bent and twisted under, and though the pressure causing this may also develop corns, and injury of the toe joint, the joint itself is not forced out of place, nor is the bad effect so common, nor so serious as in the case of the large one.

Figure 14 represents the sole of a crooked last, such as may occasionally be seen in use by some of our best boot-makers at the present time. Contrasted with the one be-

side it, which is a pretty fair specimen of right-and-left
lasts generally, it is evidently nearer to the true form.   In

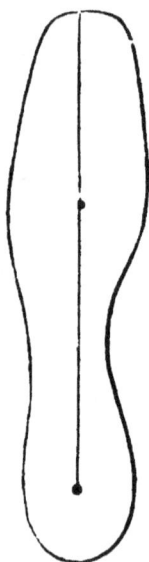

FIG. 14.—COMPROMISE.   FIG. 15.—COMMON SOLE.

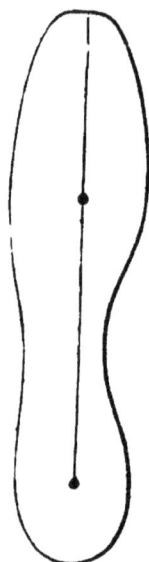

it, the line drawn from the middle of the heel to the
middle of the ball region passes through the toe nearest
the outside corner, leaving the greater space at the inside;
while in the other the line passes through the toe at the
middle, thus making it virtually only a *straight* last, hollowed out a little the most at the inner side.   For the
purpose of giving the great toe a straight position, it is
seen at a glance that the form of Fig. 14 is far superior
to that of Fig. 15, though the tendency to distortion
would still remain with it to a considerable extent.   For
the sake of a name to distinguish it, this may be called

the *Compromise*. It is not so much in advance of the common styles that many people would notice the differ-ence at all, and last-makers and shoe manufacturers might adopt it, and with a slight effort force it into general use, with great benefit to those feet that are still tolerably well-shaped, if not to their own direct advantage. At least, the acceptance of it is one step in the right direc-tion for those who are not ready to make a more radical innovation.

Our next form is something better. The reason for it is the rule given, some fifty or sixty years ago, by Dr. Peter Camper, of Amsterdam, who wrote an essay on the sub-ject, in which he stated *that the proper form of shoe was such as to allow all the toes to lie parallel with a line drawn through the middle of the sole from heel to toe.*

This, though not perfect, was, considering its date, a pretty good standard; but the shoemakers, if they were ever governed by it at all, have transgressed it since, until its intention has been entirely defeated. They have done this by narrowing the toe of the sole so much that the toes of the foot, instead of lying parallel to each other and to the line of the foot's length, have had their ends drawn together at an angle till they were compelled even to lie one over the other.

When the toes lie as closely together as they can with-out crowding—parallel, the middle ones at least, to the line of the foot's length—there is but little variation on the inside of the foot from a straight line. The cuts 16

and 17 represent, one a foot in which the toes are drawn
together just enough to touch, and one as they usually
appear in the common boot.

Here it may be observed that in Fig. 16 the lines drawn

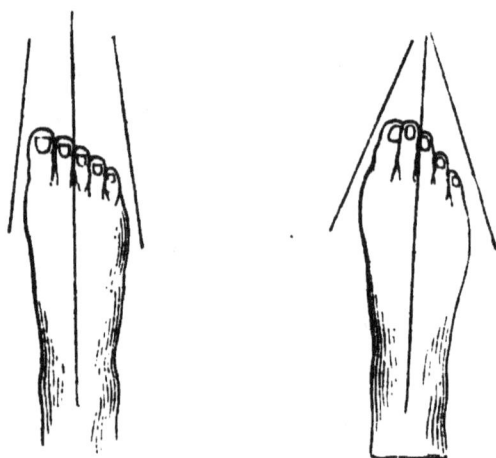

FIG. 16.—TOES PARALLEL.   FIG. 17.—TOES DRAWN TO AN ANGLE.

past the sides of the toes are nearly parallel to the line
through the foot's centre, while in Fig. 17 they quickly
form an angle with it.

Dr. Camper's rule, strictly interpreted, would have
made a right-and-left last of the most extreme character, but by narrowing the toe from inside and outside
alike, it was converted into one no better than straight.
What is now proposed is, that we take this rule and
amend it by providing *that when the inside of the sole has
the right form to let the great toe lie parallel to the line
through the middle, any further narrowing of the toe shall*

be done from the outside only; and as the ball of the last projects slightly over the bottom or sole, it is conceived that the inside margin of the *sole* should be nothing less than straight, and parallel to the line of the foot's length, from the ball forward, in order to give the great toe the position claimed. This would make a last a little more straight on the inside than the one described as the

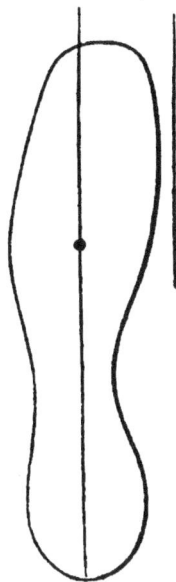

FIG. 18.—SOLE OF EXCELSIOR LAST.

Compromise. We will call it the *Excelsior*, and represent it by a diagram, Fig. 18.

Our reason for insisting that the toe be narrowed only from the outside is the fact already stated, that the consequences of bending the great toe are far worse than those of bending the little ones. Besides, it is not intended to draw them together any farther than to make them touch, and this can be done without distorting any of them, by leaving the great one in its natural position, or nearly so, and making all the curve of the sole on the outside. The outside toes being shortest, they permit this to be done without bending them more than a very little. Of course it must be remembered that the sole cannot be narrowed beyond a certain limit without injury to the foot. A medium width of toe is the narrowest that is allowable, consistently with the object we have in view.

The *last-maker* will understand that the thickest part of the toe of the last is not to be at the middle, but at the inside, in order to give room for the great toe in the straight-ahead position claimed for it. At the ball the wood is expected to project, as in all lasts, very slightly over the bottom.

This is, perhaps, the best form—the nearest approach to that of the foot—which is practically attainable while the modern boot and shoe retain their present peculiarity, of a sole narrower at the toe than at the ball. On the whole, it is probably equal or superior to that recommended by Prof. Meyer, for though his is more crooked, giving larger latitude to the great toe, it is a question if it does not, by the extreme curve, tend to cramp the little ones more than necessary, thus making a balance between a good point and a bad one. Prof. Meyer's form may be best for certain feet, and for a particular purpose, as will be explained in speaking of the remedy for crooked toes, but for general purposes we have more faith in this. If it were adopted in general use, and more especially for the shoes of children, and those who have not yet seriously deformed their feet at the joint, the next generation would show that crooked toes, soft corns, inverted nails, big joints, and bunions had been almost abolished. Such a result is entirely worthy of a noble effort on the part of those who furnish foot coverings. Such an effort, too, when made, will surely be seconded by the growing intelligence of the whole people, who will be constantly learning a better appreciation of the reform. It is to be hoped that manufacturers and wearers will both see what is for their credit and interest, and unite in securing its realization.

But it will not do to be content with what is, after all, only a rough approximation to the perfect form, for, superior as is the Excelsior last to all the existing shapes, it is still but a transition to one more complete and more permanently enduring. Like all the others, it fails to give the outside toes a chance to keep their natural form. The foot, in its normal condition, does not very closely resemble any of the shapes that have here been illustrated. It is only after it has been distorted that there appears any real fitness between it and the shoe. The forward part of the foot is wider than the middle; but this fact is not recognized in making its covering. Even Prof. Meyer is no more consistent than others, as may

be seen by contrasting one of the specimens of natural
feet which he shows us with the sole of a shoe such as
he would have it clothed with. As exhibited in the cuts
below, is there any good correspondence between the two,
except that both have a general straightness upon the
inside ?

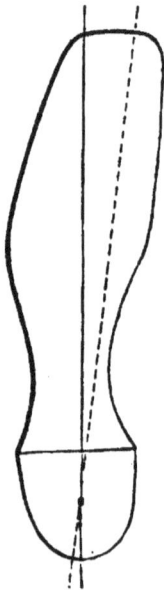

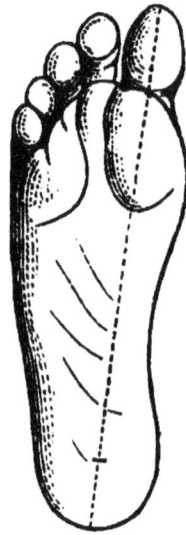

FIG. 19.—MEYER'S FORM OF SOLE.   FIG. 20.—NATURAL FOOT.

The foot is a wide one, and the shoe-sole rather narrow ; but this need not be taken into account, for the
same want of harmony would exist if the widths were
alike. A narrow foot, however, may be seen by reference
to Fig. 8, in a preceding chapter.

The only way out of this awkward inconsistency is the

acceptance of the form before suggested, and here repro-
duced (Fig. 21) to be compared with its competitors.

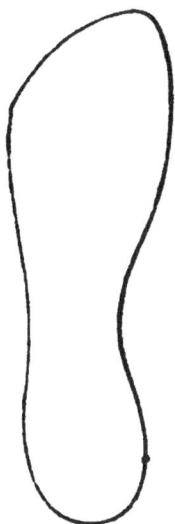

FIG. 21.—EUREKA.

This has all the merits of any of them, and the additional one that it allows as much freedom to the toes at
the *out*side of the foot as to those at the *in*side. All have
a chance, provided other things are as they should be, to
develop normally and to perform their functions without
interference. There *is* an agreement beween *it* and the
foot, not only on one side, *but on both sides and all
around.* It represents completely the idea of Dr. Camper, which cannot be done by anything of the narrow-toed
form. By a very slight addition to the width from the
ball forward, on the inside, it also represents the idea of

Prof. Meyer.   So far as we can see, it fulfils all the requirements that can be made concerning the *form of sole.*
It is proposed to name it the *Eureka.*

If a requirement were made that it should agree with the present popular taste, this pattern would signally fail. But though it does not do this, still, if it corresponds with the true form of the foot, and possesses the merits claimed, its excellence will, in time, be acknowledged, and public taste will come to see its *elegance* also.   If there is any reason at all why a thing is beautiful, that reason consists in its fitness or propriety ; and if there is any shape more fit and proper for a sole that is to be trod upon by an undeformed foot, will some one discover it and make it known.

Taste comes, at least to a great extent, from education. The teaching of China creates a taste which admires a short, stumpy, small, useless foot, as beautiful on a lady. In more enlightened countries a more intelligent taste condemns such a foot as anything else than elegant.   A still better educated taste will admire only one that is entirely normal ; and to bring opinion up to this standard is the object of effort.   People are to learn that pointed toes and big joints are not natural; that they do not come of themselves, and that the foot-gear which produces them cannot have any propriety or beauty.   The various long-toed, narrow-toed, broad-toed, stub-toed, short-heeled, thick-soled, stiff, awkward things that are worn by the masses must be seen to be, as they are, unfit

coverings to be put upon a decent human foot. Shapes,
styles, and fashions must be judged by their harmony or
want of harmony with natural requirements, and accepted
or rejected accordingly. There must be less deference to
an unreasoning, arbitrary opinion, and more of original
thought and independent action; though it could hardly
be supposed that for such a matter any great amount of
personal independence would be required. A different
set of views and tastes will thus, however, be substituted
for the present ones, as the work of time and a more general knowledge of the subject.

There is no difficulty in starting a revolutionary movement. Any of the proposed forms of lasts can be obtained
from the lastmakers of the large cities—all but the Eureka
very readily—and often the shoemaker himself, if ingenious,
can provide them for individual feet *by altering some of
those now in use.*

This is not so very difficult when the last has sufficient
thickness at the toe. At the inside, from the ball forward,
it may be shaved or rasped off enough to give a plane surface half an inch or more in width, a shoulder being cut
at the commencement near the ball. Successive layers of
firm, solid sole-leather are then pegged or nailed very
strongly to the wood without splitting it, each thickness
separately, to make the work more firm, until enough are
on to bring the corner out where it should be, when they
are rasped into the form required. Nails must not be
driven in the outside pieces. The opposite side of the toe

may be narrowed, curved, and thinned to give the whole the proper shape.

There is no reason why those persons who are capable of appreciating the doctrine of this treatise should not set an example worthy of imitation ; and as the abuses complained of are so very common, it is quite probable they might soon find themselves in the company of a large number.   Ultimately, it is expected that something not less perfect than the form last proposed, and having all the qualities desirable in a model shoe, will be universally adopted.

There will still remain to be discovered a mode of covering the foot which will secure to it all its natural freedom.   What this will be it is not easy, just now, to tell.   Possibly it may take the peculiarity of the glove, and provide separate apartments for each of the toes, becoming thus a kind of foot-glove, with a flexible sole, separated between the toes, and which will allow them to bend or spread, and the whole foot to lengthen or contract without hindrance whenever occasion may require.   It will be an article of luxury, rather than otherwise, and there is no prospect of its immediate production.   Yet such an one cannot, without difficulty, perhaps, be made sufficiently thick to be a good protection against dampness and the coldest weather.   Some compromise, with the existing style of boot will become necessary, though a shape better adapted to the comfort of the toes may be given to the forward part of it, as by the time it is made, the cramping, narrow-toed boot will be out of favour; and this brings us again to the Eureka as the most appropriate form.

What, now, can be done toward the cure of crooked toes and enlarged joints after they have been induced? The way of their prevention is already made plain, but to remove the disfigurement after it has become a settled thing is a much more difficult matter. The toe must be forced back to its former position, and kept there by a steady, constant pressure, and the parts be allowed time to gradually re-adapt themselves and grow fixed in their proper shape. The straightening of the toe will allow the bones to come nearer together at the joint, and this, when not sore, may perhaps be pushed back slightly, toward the middle of the foot, by the pressure of a narrow boot. As this process is the exact opposite of that by which the deformity is developed, it ought, with proper time, patience, and thôroughness, to be tolerably successful. Dr. Meyer even leaves it to be inferred that toes which are not badly distorted will gradually re-assume their primary position *without any assistance*, provided the shoe is of the right form, with plenty of room at the end, and the stocking is not allowed to prevent.

For straightening the toe it would seem that some efficient mechanical contrivance could be easily arranged, but as yet there is nothing entirely satisfactory. To be completely successful it ought to be something that can

4

be easily fastened to the bare foot, so that all the toes may
be brought to their proper place before covering with the
stocking.   But there is a difficulty in making the little toe,
or even more than one of them, act as a point of support
from which a force can be brought to bear against the
great one.   So, while unable to do better, this stationary
point must be found in the sole of the shoe.   The best
thing we have been able to discover is a simple plate of
metal, standing upright between the great toe and its
neighbour, so securely fastened to the insole as to prevent
the toe from inclining toward the side.   Of course nothing
can be done in a boot or shoe of the common form, as in
such a one the toe cannot be straightened by any means
whatever.   The last on which it is made must be one like
that described as the *Excelsior*, or, what is still better for
this case, one of the form proposed by Dr. Meyer.   There
is no danger of going to an extreme in so shaping the last
as to turn the toe inward, because, the toe, after being fastened at its end, tends strongly to resume its old, deformed
position by pushing the upper over the edge of the sole at
the joint.   It thus partially defeats the object, and will be
straightened less than the form of the last (and shoe) indicates that it ought to be.   Hence it is well not to let the
ball of the last project over the bottom, and thus try to
keep back the joint from pushing over the upper of the
shoe.   And, even if the last is crooked inward at the toe
a little *more* than Meyer's rule directs, there will be no
harm.   It should also be well hollowed or curved on the

inside, at the region back of the ball and above the shank. The more the wood is taken off here, the more the foot will be thrown toward the outside of the shoe, or made to tread outside, and this will somewhat counterbalance the tendency which the toe has, when the end of it is made stationary, to push the joint and whole foot toward the inside. The crookedness will appear extreme, and perhaps ridiculous, but it will be found in practice that it takes a *very* crooked shoe to make a big toe straight.

We believe, however, that this tendency of the toe and joint to keep their old position by treading over inside can be counteracted by putting a low counter or stiffening of sole-leather into the upper of the shoe at the ball, in the same way a similar one is inserted at the heel. Or, if the joint is too sensitive to be touched by stiff leather, let the stiffening piece be placed just back of the ball, in the shank. The top part of it must be thinned, while the bottom part remains thick and firm. It has not been fairly tried, but if the joint is not sore it can hardly fail to be effective.

It should be a *false* insole to which the partition or separator is fastened, so that it can be easily changed, because there is some difficulty in fitting it exactly right the first time, and, besides, the wearer may wish, even when it suits as well as possible, to remove it and give the toe a resting-spell in its old position ; while if the partition is secured to the proper insole of the boot, it must remain

4—2

there, whether right or wrong, and in the latter case the boot will be worthless.

A strip of *thick tin*, half or three-fourths of an inch wide, and two and a half inches long, is all that is required for the material. If preferred, it may be of thin sheet iron or sheet brass. Any tinsmith will furnish it, bent and doubled into the form represented in the diagram.

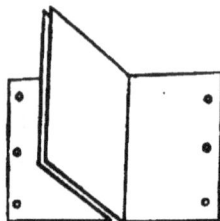

FIG. 22.—SEPARATOR.

The upright part is five-eighths or three-fourths of an inch high, according to the thickness of the toes. A cut is made in the insole, and this part put through, while the ends are fastened to the under-side of the sole by some very small-headed tacks, such as every shoemaker has upon his bench, or can readily procure, and can drive after making holes through the tin with a sharp-pointed peg-awl, clinching their points on his lap-iron ; or if the part goes through snugly, there is no real need of fastening at all. It is best not to set the partition very far back from the end of the toe, because at the first joint there is but a thin covering of flesh to guard the bone from being hurt. The exact place for it must be determined by carefully measuring the foot, *while the toe is kept straight* by the hand, and afterward measuring the same length on the insole, with the size-stick ; the *width* of the toe, as well as the foot's length, being also taken, and in the same way. To make sure that it shall not chafe the toe, the partition or separator may be covered neatly with cloth, or with a piece of thin sheepskin or kid leather. The following cut shows it when ready to be put into the shoe.

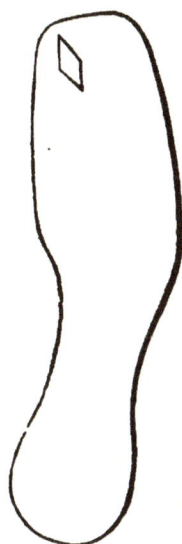

FIG. 23.—INSOLE WITH SEPARATOR.

The edges and corners of the separator need to be smoothly rounded, and the forward upright corner may be lowered by filing off, if desired, to prevent its showing against the upper. It should not be *wider* or thicker at its forward part, that is, it should not be triangular-shaped,* so as to separate the toes more at the ends than farther back, for if so it would prevent the smaller ones from straightening out to correspond with the large one. The large toe often pushes the smaller ones to the outside —part of them, at least—and when the great toe is restored to straightness the smaller ones should be allowed to follow it, as they will be inclined to do, while the curve of the shoe on the outside tends also to push them back toward the inside. Almost anything between them will keep them apart temporarily, as for the purpose of giving ease to a sore joint, where there is no intention to continue the improvement.

When the shoe is made ready there may still be some difficulty about getting the foot into it. There must first be a toe made in the stocking; which can be done in a rough way by sewing two parallel seams, an eighth of an inch or so apart, from the end of the stocking to a depth equal to the length of the great toe, of sufficient width to give room for it, and then cutting down between these seams with the scissors. The stocking should itself be of

---

* There is no objection to this form in particular cases where it is desired to go to an extreme in straightening the toe, provided that side of the separator next the small toes be kept straight, and the increase of width made to throw the great one still farther inward. It may be done by filing off the forward corner of the upright portion till its two sides are separated nearly back to the opposite corner, when a wedge of leather can be inserted to keep them apart. There must be plenty of room in the upper, or the pressure of such a separator may create soreness at the nail. .

good width, to give space for the smaller toes to be separated also. An ingenious woman would probably find a better way of making the toe, but this will answer if necessary. Then, if the joint is not too stiff, or the toe too much bent aside, it can be kept straight while going into the boot by the fingers of one hand pressing against it outside of the upper leather; and when this is the case the foot may be clothed in any kind of a boot or shoe, and no difficulty will be experienced in putting it on. A man's calf boot may be drawn on in this way the first time it is worn.

But when the deformity is too decided to allow of the toe being kept straight by the hand in this manner, a shoe *which laces in front* must be made, the opening being cut down *somewhat lower than usual*—as low, in fact, as will answer—though the line of the vamp is still curved so much that the seam will not cross the joints—a direction which the maker will understand. On account of the vamp being so short, the shoe will look better if made rather long for the foot.

With this the foot can be turned a little, and worked around in such a way as commonly to get the toe to go in on the right side of the partition ; but if there is still difficulty, a pretty sure way of accomplishing the object is to take a yard of tape, ribbon, or something similar, wind it up around the finger into a large, compact wad, and crowd it in between the toes till the great one is well straightened out, taking care to leave one end of the tape hanging outside the shoe. The toe will then be likely to go into the place made for it, and the tape can be pulled out by its free end before the shoe is fully drawn on.

A low shoe is still better than a high one for these difficult cases, as the lower it is the more freedom will be allowed to turn the foot one side in entering the toe.

Even where no trouble of this kind is anticipated, it is still advisable that the first trial be made with a laced shoe —whether high or low is not material—when, if entirely successful, a boot, or a Button gaiter may next be ventured ; and to those who cannot feel sufficient faith in these statements to risk a failure on a pair of good shoes, we recommend that they have a pair made of the poorest and cheapest materials, and try them as an experiment.

᛫ The methods here given of straightening the toe, and the way of making the shoe and getting the foot into it, have been tried with fair success. Great toes that were badly deformed have been brought back so much as to give the appearance of well-formed feet, without creating any discomfort, and with positive ease and benefit to all the other toes. Of course, the less the distortion, and the less time it has existed, the easier to accomplish the purpose. There may be many cases which there would be little use in attempting to reform ; but the great majority can probably be improved ; and though a complete success may not be always attainable, the gain in appearance, to say nothing of comfort, ought to be sufficient inducement to make a trial of the plan.

In some cases an unpleasant feeling to the toe or joint may be occasioned by the change, as might be expected in any change of a similar kind, but it is likely to become less and less till it entirely disappears.

The greatest direct benefit, however, will doubtless be in the case of bunion or other soreness of the joint, where the straightening of the toe would give immediate relief, and furnish a motive to continue the new habit. The difficulty of effecting this in the common-shaped shoe is well known to those who have had occasion to try it. With the new form it will be comparatively easy.

Having the great toe corrected, and the smaller ones left free to correct themselves, being also influenced to do so by the curve on the outside of the shoe, there is the best reason to believe that by perseveringly continuing the position for a sufficient length of time, all the parts would return permanently to their natural form. In the worst cases this time might be several years; in others only as many months. The law that any limb or organ of the body will adapt itself to a change of position is one that cannot be questioned; the only doubt is as to the extent of the change which may be thus effected. When the foot has been years in growing into a bad shape, it cannot be expected to right itself immediately, though much may depend upon the thoroughness with which the remedy is applied.

Prevention, however, is said to be far better than cure. It certainly is in this matter, and, being so easy and simple, there can hardly be any good reason for its neglect.

As a means of developing some hints that may be of service in originating an article superior to any now worn, as well as a matter of curiosity, and to show some of the elegance formerly existing, we give a few representations

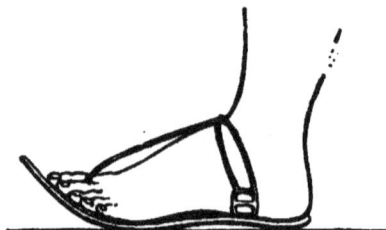
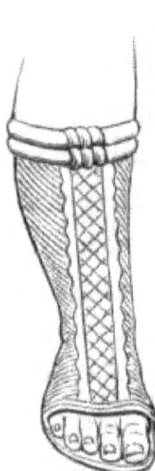
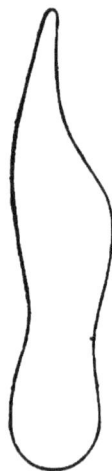

FIG. 24. FIG. 25. FIG. 26.

ANCIENT EGYPTIAN. ROMAN. OLD ENGLISH

of the foot-apparel worn in ancient and medieval times. It seems possible there may be some peculiarity about them that can be adopted and made of use for the future. We are indebted for them to Mr. J. S. Hall's "BOOK OF THE FEET."

The first cut is that of a sandal worn by the aristocracy of Egypt in the earliest ages. There is a fastening over the instep, and another passing from that, to a point between the great toe and the smaller ones, to prevent slipping toward either side. The foot is a handsome one —evidently that of a lady—and the sandal seems appropriate to a dry, warm climate, in the days when a partially bare foot had not become disgraceful.

The second figure represents the *cothurnus* of the old Romans—a sort of boot-sandal, laced in front down to the roots of the toes, but leaving the toes themselves exposed and free, and with a sole like a sandal, evidently shaped to fit the foot—not the foot to fit *it*. The sturdy conquerors of the world did not, it is plain, believe in subjecting their toes to any such tyranny as we impose upon ours. Who can say the foot is not finely formed, although the toes are not drawn together into a pile? or that the covering is not appropriate, neat, and elegant?

Figure 26 shows us a form of shoe in fashion among the nobility of England in the fifteenth century. Though the toe is somewhat lengthy, the shoe is otherwise eminently sensible. We ought to be, and think we are, able to improve upon what was done by our ancestors of four hundred years ago ; yet here is a sole that, notwithstanding its ridiculously long toe, is better adapted to fit the natural foot and preserve its shape than any of those made at the present day. A turn-up toe is not so objectionable, when of moderate length, as it leaves less necessity for a high heel. And if our shoes must have long and narrow toes, something like this is decidedly *better*, and no more ridiculous, than the cramping, distorting shapes now in use. It is at least extraordinary that with all our modern wisdom we are not yet able to produce a better form than any of them. But while waiting for the right thing, if the Paris *cordonniers* will adopt this, and return it to us duly indorsed as the latest orthodox French style, there will be reason for gratitude to them, and for congratulation among ourselves.

It may be noticed that the form here shown would, if its long toe were taken off, have a strong resemblance to that called the *Eureka*, the breadth at the part where the toes lie, being its best and most important point. And thus comparing the Eureka with all the *modern* shapes of boots and shoes, we are compelled to re-assert that it is not only the best of any for all proper purposes, but that, looked upon with a rightly educated taste—with a knowledge that the forward part of the foot is, and ought to be, the widest—it is also the most beautiful.

CHAPTER V.

Flattened Condition of the Arch—Beauty of one that is Natural—
Nature and Purpose of its Construction—How it Becomes Broken
Down—Lengthening of the Foot—Lack of Development—Means
of Improvement—Lasts for Flat Feet—Transverse Arch.

ANOTHER of the prominent disfigurements of the
foot is that commonly known as *flat-foot*, which is
seen where the arch of the instep is in a broken-down or
flattened condition. This deformity has, if possible, a
more awkward and ungraceful effect than that caused by
the unnatural position of the toes and joints ; though there
may be less painful effects attending it than are attached
to the latter. The worst trouble accompanying this kind
of disfigurement is the *weakness* which is attendant upon
it, and which is sometimes so extreme as to interfere
seriously with walking for any great distance, or standing
long at a time ; making itself felt at various periods, as
there happens to be a demand for strength and activity.

It is almost needless to say how unnatural is such a
condition. Children are seldom subject to it, except when

connected with weak ankles. Even the children of parents who are notoriously flat-footed have feet that are tolerably well arched. We venture to say that the wild Indian of the native forest was never seen with the beauty of his symmetrical and handsome frame marred by flat feet. There are some of the race who flatten their *heads*, but they never wear boots, nor heels on their moccasins, and their feet are therefore free from this disagreeable shape. The artist never allows a representation of this deformity to appear in his work ; on the contrary, an arch that is high and well-marked has always been considered beautiful. It gives an airiness, elegance, and grace to the appearance of the foot which is as beautiful as the flat foot is ungraceful and awkward. A firm step and upright carriage of the whole body are also generally to be found with the arched instep—never without ; while the flat foot, if not seen, may always be inferred from the unnatural, shuffling gait of its possessor.

The high arch is thus beautiful for the same reason that any other organ or part of the body is beautiful—because it is better adapted to perform its intended function or office, which is the support of the weight of the body, this design being more perfectly accomplished when the arch is high, because it is then stronger than when low or flattened. To flatten it is like drawing apart the ends upon which it rests, and this, it is apparent, weakens, if it does not entirely break, the unity and strength of the whole.

The nature of the construction of the foot in this respect is thus set forth by Prof. Meyer :

" If the inner aspect of the foot is examined, we find that it is an arch, resting in front on the anterior heads of the five metatarsal bones, but principally on that of the great toe, and on that of the calcaneum behind. The astragalus forms the key-stone of the arch.

" The arch is enabled to retain its form by means of strong ligaments or bands passing from one bone to the others, and thus held closely together, sustains the super-incumbent weight of the body without giving way.

" When we rest on the foot, as in standing, the arch is flattened by the pressure from above, and consequently becomes *lengthened*. When, however, the foot is allowed to hang free, *the curvature of the arch is increased.* At every step in walking, also, when the foot is raised from the ground, *the curvature immediately becomes greater through the action of the muscles.*"

This action, it will be readily seen, is precisely that of a spring under a carriage, or other similar vehicle, and seems to have a like intention—that of preventing the transmission of a shock or jar to the joints, and the internal organs of the body above.

It will be found true, we believe, that in persons of mus-cular temperament—the temperament that gives tall, spare, and angular forms—the curvature of the arch is greater than in those whose natural disposition of body is toward fleshiness. In the latter case, the muscles of the whole system being weaker, they allow the bones of the foot to separate more easily, and this, consequently, allows the flattening.   In other words, we strongly suspect that in this temperament of the body the ligaments are not so dense, firm, and strong as they are in persons whose physical structure is more predominantly muscular.   The ligaments which hold the bones together at the joints are not designed to stretch, under ordinary circumstances, but they do yield when sufficient force is exerted upon them, as in the case of sprains and dislocations, and it is reasonable to infer that they adapt themselves to the demand made upon them.   The muscles grow longer and larger, as do also the bones, under circumstances that call for such growth or adaptations to conditions.   So do *all* the organs and tissues of the body, in greater or less degree ; and if the ligaments do not, they are a plain exception, which is not probable.   This being so, a constant strain upon the ligaments of the foot's arch, as in standing for several hours without rest, must cause them to stretch somewhat, allowing the bones to loosen and sink down, while the same severe strain, if continued for a yet longer period, would force them to grow into this lengthened condition, to meet the demand upon them, thus rendering the fault permanent.   In persons of fleshy tendency, the natural softness and weakness of the muscles and ligaments allow them the more easily to give way to the pressure upon the arch.   It is believed to be the fact that the deformity is more common among people of this type, and it will be well for those so constituted to guard against anything that tends to its development.

It is in persons of the opposite type—those who have firm, close, hard, and strong muscles, and no extra flesh— that the arch is found in its greatest perfection. There the strong muscles and ligaments bind the bones together with such firmness that the arch is enabled longer to resist the influences which tend to break it down. Yet the flat foot is very common, in spite of all nature's efforts for prevention. The deformity, in greater or less degree, may be said to exist as the rule among adult persons, while the natural arch is the exception. Among some classes of people, flat-foot is almost wholly prevalent. Hard toil and degrading conditions not only debase the person morally and intellectually, but they affect the gait and carriage, and their influence may be seen to reach down to the very bottom of the foot.

It was this fault, possibly, which first suggested the practice of wearing heels, or, if it did not originate, at least continued it. *Heels partially restore that elevation and airiness of the foot which is given by a natural arch,* and which constitutes its grace and beauty. When rightly made, and worn as a choice of two evils, or as a partial remedy for an evil, they are not objectionable; but they can be only a partial corrective. They can never be sub- stituted for a good arch; while, worn as they are and have · been, *they really become one of the causes* of the deformity

5

which in turn calls for their use.   Another cause is thus
explained in Prof. Meyer's book :

"Flat-foot is occasioned by the loosening of the ligaments that knit the foot firmly together, and, by the consequent sinking of the arch, the inner aspect of the foot
no longer presents the natural hollow in the sole.   The
causes of such loosening of the ligaments are numerous,
but by far the most frequent, and one readily induced by
the ordinary shoe, is weight improperly directed on the
arch.   If, for example, a shoe happens to be trodden on one side, and especially, as is most commonly
the case, if it be so at the heel, then the heel has no support, except from the inner margin of the sole, which is
thus worn away, and the heel-piece becomes oblique, or,
in other words, lower at one side than the other.   In walking and standing on such a heel-piece, the whole external
margin of the foot is raised, and the inner, which naturally
supports the arch, is so depressed as gradually to lose its
convexity, and thus flat-foot is produced."

The nature of the cause here spoken of seems to be
like that of a *sprain*, to a slight degree, and may be an
influential one, but we doubt that it is the most common
cause of that loosening of the ligaments which allows the
foot to break down.   The most common and efficient of
all the causes of this difficulty, it appears to us, is the
short heel which has always been worn on boots and shoes,
and is still, except where an innovation upon its shape has
been made within a few years past.   This, though not

strictly a direct cause, like a strain from above, is the condition which most frequently admits and encourages the sinking of the arch.

That *short heels* most frequently admit of and encourage the sinking of the arch of the foot will be readily seen by an explanation. There are several bones which, together, form the forward part of the arch, while the back part consists of one larger bone, technically called the *calcaneum*, or *os calcis*, which makes up the principal part of the heel. Partly above this, and between it and the forward bones, is the one called the *astragalus*, which is the keystone, being located the highest of any, and the one upon which rest the bones of the leg; in size it is next to the *calcaneum*. An illustration will show the position.

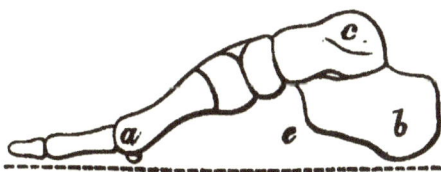

FIG. 27.

The inner aspect of the foot, showing the arched construction of the whole foot—*a*, head of metatarsal bone of great toe,—*b*, calcaneum,—*c*, astragalus.

The forward part of the *calcaneum*, or heel-bone, at its lower surface, is somewhat higher than the back part, and has under it a thicker cushion of flesh. When the bare foot treads upon the surface, or when there is no heel upon the shoe-sole, this point—letter *e* in the diagram—is as well supported as any other, and, being so, enables all the other bones to keep their proper places, but when there is a heel on the sole of the shoe, it *is not long enough—does not extend under far enough*—to support this *forward part* of the heel-bone. The sole, forward of the heel, is not usually stiff enough to support it, and therefore it falls downward as much as the leather will give way; the heel-piece being often half an inch too short, and sometimes more than that. Then, if the sole is light, so as to give way easily, there is nothing to prevent this part of the bone from settling down to the extent of a quarter of an inch, or even more. While the back part is supported, the front is turning directly downward. This allows the astragalus and the whole arch to sink down to the same extent, and, in time, all parts of the foot will adapt themselves to their changed condition, and the flat shank become a permanent thing. If any person will examine a slipper worn with a heel, or a *boot* having an ordinary sole, it will be seen that just in front of the heel the sole is depressed, or bent downward, from one-eighth to three-eighths of an inch. This is almost invariable, except when a very long heel, or a stiff shank in the sole, preserves the natural position of the *calcaneum* or bone of which the heel is formed. The amount of this depression shows how much the arch has sunk, and how much higher it would be if properly supported. It indicates very plainly the occasion and origin of a large proportion of the flat and splay feet that may be so frequently observed.

This inefficiency of the common short heel to properly

support the arch was first discovered by Dr. J. C. Plumer, of Boston, to whom is due the credit of showing the bad offoots just noticed as the result of its being worn. His style of boot and last will be discussed further on.

It has been stated that as the foot flattens, it also lengthens. It has been estimated that some flat feet are as much as two sizes, or two-thirds of an inch, longer than the same feet would be if well arched; an item worth noticing by those who are fastidious upon this point.

In falling down, the *calcaneum* is pushed backward making the long-heeled foot, while the bones forward of the *astragalus* must advance more or less in *their* direction, thus adding to the foot's length at both ends, and making the leg appear to be set far toward the middle. The ends must necessarily be separated before the middle of the arch can sink, and this is why its flattening is accompanied by the long heel. In a foot that is well arched, the projection of bone at the upper part of the heel extends farther back than the lower edge at the sole. In a flat foot, on the contrary, the bottom part extends back farther than the bony projection above, which, in fact, is pretty sure not to project at all.

It may be asked, Why not keep the ends of the arch together by a boot that is short at both ends, supposing such a one could be made that would not distort the toes? Simply because it would prevent the *use*, and consequent *strength*, of the muscles of the under side of the foot, *which are themselves the natural bands for holding the ends together*, and the whole arch in its raised position. These muscles, being weakened by the cramping of a short boot, would allow the arch to sink whenever the artificial support was taken away. This reasoning seems to indicate such a treatment as one of the causes by which flatness is produced, and as pinching the foot lengthwise has been a common fault, this cause may have been quite effective.

Dr. Meyer thus refers to another bad influence :

"We have already seen that the foot forms an arch, *the efficiency of which in a special manner depends on the tensity of its ligaments being maintained. If then, an unnatural and flattening pressure be constantly exercised on this arch, the binding ligaments get slackened and the arch falls down ;* a broken-down arch, as we have already seen, causes flat-foot. The pressure of the upper leather on the instep must, therefore, and particularly in the case of narrow boots, favour the origin of this deformity. The same cause must further interfere with locomotion, for at every step the increased arching of the instep, which takes place the moment that the foot is set to [? raised from] the ground is resisted by the upper leather, and an injurious influence is thus exercised on the action of some of the muscles used in walking, and which runs from the anterior aspect of the lower leg to the back of the foot."

All cramping, binding, and confining of *any part of the body* weakens it, as is well known to every intelligent reader. Hence the manifest impropriety of wearing anything unnecessarily tight or binding to the arch of the instep. Every boot that is uncomfortably tight has to some degree the effect of weakening, and rendering it more liable to fall down.

More especially is this the case when the leather used is *thick, hard,* or *stiff*. Much of the cheap and inferior goods offered for sale ready-made are seriously objectionable on this account. The uppers themselves are—a large share of them, at least—thick and hard, while the pegged soles are made as stiff as possible, to give the appearance of thick, solid, and serviceable leather in that part. Many a poor man is thus actually hobbled, to a greater or less extent, by the miserable foot-gear his poverty compels him to wear. As there is but very little *bend* to them, *there is but little use of the muscles of the foot.* It is cramped or unnaturally pressed upon, even though having plenty of room, and might almost as well be cased in iron as in the stiff kip or cowhide boot or brogan. The result is weakness, flattening, and a tendency to other kinds of distortion. We believe the frequency of flat-foot among some of the poorer classes of people may thus be easily accounted for.

The peasantry of other countries are even less fortunate than our own. Saying nothing of wooden shoes, the leather ones they wear are not only thick and stiff in material, but the soles are often filled with stout iron nails besides. With such things on the feet there can be no spring to the toes, no use for the forward part of the arch, no play to the muscles.   The feet can hardly be otherwise than weak and flat.   When tightness is added to stiffness the effect must be still worse.

Children must feel these bad consequences more than adults, for being less firm in their muscles and bones, they have less power of resisting the cramping, weakening influence.   Some of the boots manufactured in this country for boys can be recommended only as a slightly less evil than going barefoot in cold weather.

One other reason is, very probably, *lack of development*. The calf of the leg is but partially developed in some races of men, and only comes to its full growth in conditions of civilized society that call for the use of all its muscles.   So it is confidently believed that all those steps and motions which give lightness, grace, ease, and elegance to the movements of the body, such as occur in most varieties of the dance, *and particularly such as demand the use of the toes*, have a tendency to develop and strengthen the foot's arch.   As *its* full development tends to créate easy, light, and graceful movements, *so these in turn help it to grow into full strength and beauty*. Hence the well-developed calf, the well-arched foot, and the graceful step will almost invariably be found to go together.

There may be yet other and unknown causes of this deformity ; but enough have been noticed to account for the great majority of cases.   While it is already very common, the influences that have produced it are still

producing and confirming the wrong shape. Of course
the longer the fault is established the more difficult it is
to make a change; but there is believed to be a partial
remedy, at least, in the case of young persons. It consists
in simply supporting the back part of the arch as nature
does in her own way; that is, in supporting the whole
under-surface of the calcaneum, or heel-bone, as is done
when the bare foot is pressed upon the ground. A long
heel—one extending under the sole far enough for its front
edge to support the front part of the bone—is the thing
required. When the foot rests upon such a heel, the
whole weight of the body acts as a force to compel the
forward part of the bone to push itself upward into its
true place, because, being a quarter of an inch—more or
less—lower than it ought to be, it cannot be perfectly at
ease until it gets back where it belongs. The weight of
the body, then, is just as influential in restoring the arch
to its natural form when the long heel is worn, as it is in
breaking it down when the short heel is the only support.
There is reason to think that a large number of the flat
feet could be corrected by this simple expedient. The
long-standing cases might require considerable time, and
even prove too obdurate for this remedy; but the law
which compels all parts of the system to adapt themselves
to circumstances would tend constantly and strongly to
bring about the effect desired. In those cases where the
feet have not grown into a positive, settled distortion, we
doubt not the result would be decided and very gratifying;

and if the children wore these long heels—if, in short, the whole people were educated to see the necessity of wearing them, when any at all are worn, the instances of flat-foot would be far less common.

A few years since, Dr. Plumer (before referred to) patented a style of boot, of which the long heel is one characteristic. This is, in fact, the best thing about his invention, and should go far to make it popular, even if it has no other recommendation. The fashion has been considerably introduced in some places, and has also had some effect in increasing the length of heels in work not made after that style, and thus may indirectly have saved many from having the arch of their feet broken down. For this it is deserving of praise, though we attach less importance to its other peculiarities.

The old-fashioned way of making heels leaves them from one-fourth to five-eighths of an inch too short. The whole tendency of such heels is downward, in a double sense. The more they are worn the farther downward goes the foot, not only in *form*, but in *character*—in beauty, gracefulness, and strength.

The long heel, on the contrary, tends to raise the foot upward in shape, and also to restore its strength and grace. As a means of prevention, it should be adopted for all children, to preserve the shape of feet that are still natural.

The Plumer heel has frequently been carried to an extreme, and in such a way as to make its shape appear clumsy and inelegant. For this there is no real necessity. A heel that will extend under the foot half an inch farther than the generality of short ones, *can be made, by pitching it well under behind, to appear only slightly longer than common* at the top, (or bottom,) and be tasteful in every particular. The form may be that of the most approved, and there is no demand for greater width. If the counters or stiffenings be of the right kind, the heel may be made sufficiently narrow to look well, and correspond with the general appearance of an elegant boot, without danger of its treading over. This latter kind of trouble comes mainly from *counters that are too weak*, though, of course, a heel that is too small relatively—which is not handsome—or that is built inclining to one side, will be likely to produce the same result.

A *high* heel has an influence in encouraging this false condition of the arch by throwing the foot forward, thus creating the same effect as a shortening of the heel itself. This is not so great a cause as some others, it is true, but, as one thing tending to the same general result, it should be considered and guarded against.

It is claimed that a necessity exists for a heel of some kind in order to prevent the stubbing of the toes in walking; and the fact that people of Eastern countries turn up the toes of their shoes seems to countenance the claim. Yet, it is doubtful. Although Nature did not put anything under our heels, it cannot be supposed that she intended us to go about constantly stubbing our toes. If there had really been a need of raising up the heel, she would have raised it. It is more likely that by wearing heels we have got the foot into a false habit of pointing the toes downward more than is natural, and hence our inclination to stub them when the artificial heels are not under us, if such is the fact. The heels must be decided (described) as unnatural as they are unnecessary. Still, a moderately high one is not so obnoxious as to be worth disputing about. If the height were limited to an inch for the heels of a lady's boot, and an inch and a quarter for those of gentlemen, as a general rule, in both cases, the disadvantage of such heels would be so trifling that they could hardly be objectionable, provided the length was sufficient. But a *short* heel, however *low* it may be, is a villainous thing.

Another great means, both of preventing the fall of the arch, and of restoring it afterward—one hardly inferior to that of the heel—is the exercise and development of the muscles of the under side of the foot. These are chiefly concerned in the use of the toes. They act whenever we spring upon the forward part of the foot in walking, leaping, or dancing. Their exercise not only strengthens *them*, but it strengthens all the other parts also; the ligaments and bones, as well, being made more dense, firm, and enduring, according to the law that the proper use of the muscles of any part of the body draws blood, vitality, and strength into the surrounding or contiguous parts. As these muscles extend in a general lengthwise direction, their strong and firm condition tends directly to hold the ends of the arch as near together as they naturally belong, or in other words, prevent their separation. And as they must ˙separate before the arch can sink, it is seen that here is a powerful influence naturally exerting itself to restrain the foot from flattening; a view which can be sustained by good anatomical and medical authority.

The ladies of Spain are said to possess the finest feet of any race of women in the world. The fact can hardly be disputed; and to account therefore it is only necessary to take into consideration the general prevalence of their national habit of *dancing*, which, by all its movements and exercises of the foot, tends directly toward strength-ening the toes and raising the arch. A person who can support the weight of the body on the tips of the great toes, either naturally or by cultivation, must possess not only strong muscles in the toes themselves, but a strong arch, and strong foot throughout. We will risk the reputation of this book on the assertion that a broken-down arch cannot be found in the whole dancing *pro-fession.*

Here, then, is indicated one course of practical effort by which to avoid or ameliorate the deformity. All those movements of gymnastics which go to strengthen the foot may likewise be adopted with advantage. The toes must also be taught to do their share in the process of walking; and whatever action, in short, will cause the exercise of the muscles of the lower part of the foot, should be favoured, and will help to develop and raise the arch. But this effect cannot be produced immediately.   It may require patience, determination, and steady perseverance. There is no royal road to recovery from flat-footedness, any more than there is to knowledge.

The coverings for flat feet should always be made upon lasts that are flat in the shank like themselves. A boot made on an arched last cannot possibly fit a foot whose sole is convex from heel to toe; hence such feet need lasts made expressly for them. The upper leather of the boot cannot, in this case, be too soft and pliable. It should be loose enough to allow the bending at the ball and the movements of the toes to be performed with ease. All the muscles must have a chance to act freely, and the blood be permitted to circulate without hindrance. At the same time there is no need of having big wrinkles, or any extra looseness in the fit of the boot, if only sufficient care is taken in the making.

Another thing to be considered is the stiffening in the shank of boots, more particularly in those of men. If a short heel *must* be worn a stiff shank had better go with it. A metallic shank, if strong, will then be useful, and perhaps generally effective in keeping up the foot. A shank-piece of leather is seldom so stiff but that a flat foot will bend it downward to adapt it to its own shape. So it will also depress the steel shank at the forward and middle portions, but probably not directly in front of the heel, where the most support is required. The shank,

:oo, unless nearly straight, will be apt to press against the middle of the arch—or where the arch ought to be—so strongly as to cause discomfort; and it is a question if such a pressure does not itself tend to weaken the foot still more. It is thus doubtful if the metallic shank will be of any benefit to a flat foot, unless pains are taken to make it conform to a flat-bottomed last by straightening. Feet that are tolerably well-arched can wear it with no difficulty.

But, further: the stiffness in the shank of the boot interferes somewhat with the flexibility of the foot, and therefore no more of it than is necessary to pull off the boot ought to be allowed. By far the best way, and the only right way, is to wear a heel sufficiently long to give all the needed support, and a shank as flexible as it can be without breaking or clinging to the foot when the boot is drawn off. The foot—at least the heel and arch portion —is then left unimpeded in its natural action. If it be said that the stiffness is intended to keep the sole in its proper shape, it is replied that when the boot fits naturally and easily—not loosely—it will keep its correct shape without any help, while if it does not it will tread badly in spite of all the stiffness.

There is an additional elegance, and general appearance of elevation given to the foot by having the sole of the boot made as thin and light in the shank or waist as possible. This can be done in men's boots by driving a row of pegs through the shank-piece, putting the pegs close together, to create stiffness, without increasing the thickness of the leather. The shoemaker will understand. A shank made in this manner will be firm enough in drawing off the boot, the thickly-driven pegs not leaving room between them for the leather to *break;* while it is much more flexible than a thick one. It is thus *better adapted to the foot,* at the same time that it is *quite as reliable for its own proper purpose.* One piece of leather may thus take the place of two or three. Where a metallic shank is used, there will of course be the appearance of lightness.

The model boot or shoe of the future, however, will be one in which there shall exist no need of stiffness in order to draw it off, but where this part of the sole will be so thin and flexible as to be easily pressed downward by the large ligament under the arch when the toes are raised, while it will cling upward close to the hollow of the foot when the arch is raised and the toes extended.

Another hint to the bootmaker may not be inappropriate. It is generally considered desirable to have the side seams correspond with, or meet, the forward corners of the heel. To effect this when a long heel is made it is only necessary to add half an inch, or more, to the width of the *back-pattern* at the bottom, before cutting. This width may be added at the bottom, and lessened gradually toward the top, or continued through the whole length of the pattern equally, as preferred. A corresponding amount must of course be taken off from the width of the *front* pattern at the same time. In a boot without side-seams the same rule applies in cutting the ends of the outside counter.

The front of the heel should not be cut out in curved form, as is sometimes done, because that is a virtual shortening of it; though there is no objection to cutting out the upper lifts of the leather, letting the point of the knife come out before touching the sole, which makes a shortened appearance without affecting the length at all where the sole and heel surfaces unite. A heel *rounded out*, lengthwise, would be preferable to one curved *in*, though it might not be thought so elegant unless indorsed by fashion. We speak thus particularly about the con-struction of the heel, because it is important; as the good or ill form of the foot's arch seems to depend upon it more than upon anything else, except it be the strengthening of the muscles.

There is a third peculiarity of the Plumer last that is worthy of notice, and which consists in a hollowing out or concaving of the bottom or sole from the heel forward to the toe, but mostly through the ball. This hollow is de-signed to be filled up with leather in making the boot, so as to leave the bottom of the sole *flat*, while *inside it is rounded upward*. The object of this change in the shape of the last is to make it conform to the shape of the foot, which it does very closely. But, at the same time, so far as this has any effect upon the foot at all it has an injurious

6

one. The form of the sole of the foot at this place is one
that *ought not to be conformed to* by the sole of the boot.
There is a low arch, transversely of the foot, from the
ball of the great toe to that of the little one, its two opposite resting points. In nature it is somewhat like the
great arch between the ball and heel. To raise the
sole under it is like supporting an arch in the middle,
which would be absurd. In this case it is entirely unnatural, and only of use *in a boot that is very tight, or
much too narrow, where it may do good by preventing the
formation of a big wrinkle in the sole of the foot, lengthwise*, which might come from the drawing together of the
opposite sides. The following quotation strongly sets
forth the impropriety of the new mode.

"There has been a good deal said of late about the
transverse arch of the foot, and the necessity of supporting it to prevent its breaking down, and the unfortunate
possessor becoming splay-footed. Did any one ever hear
of an arch requiring support? * * * What is called the
transverse arch is in reality a portion of an elliptic spring;
and the moment you fill up the natural hollow of the foot
you destroy its elasticity. What carriage-maker puts supports under the arches of his carriage-springs? The
human foot is a combination of bones and strong muscles
that act as springs, and at each point where it comes in
contact with the ground is placed a cushion to prevent
jarring. When the weight of the body is placed upon the
foot, it spreads both in *length* and *breadth*, and it contracts

again when the weight is removed; and any artificial support under the hollow of the foot *prevents this expansion and contraction,* and one may as well have a wooden foot, for all practical purposes, as one which has a support under the transverse arch."*

As the foot spreads at every step, the arch naturally flattens in the middle, but this is prevented when the sole is built up under it. *It is self-evident that the foot is designed to tread on a flat surface, as its most natural function.* Any attempt to make it tread constantly on a *convex* one is manifestly wrong. Yet, as said before, it may be of use to prevent a greater evil where people are determined to wear tight or narrow boots in spite of all reason or propriety.

It is also true that a slight hollow will exist under the ball of a well-arched foot, even when pressed upon by the weight of the body. This may be filled up if desired, for, being so small, it is a matter of indifference whether it is so or not, while there is perfect safety in letting it alone.

We see, then, that while one characteristic of the Plumer boot—the long heel—is a very valuable one, another —that of filling under the transverse arch—is useless, or positively injurious. The first, or good quality, however, overbalances the latter, and therefore the boot is an improvement upon the old or common style. The true and

---

' * This paragraph is from Mr. J. L. Watkins, a boot and shoe manufacturer of New York city, who has attempted to carry into practice the idea of Prof. Meyer.

natural-shaped boot would have a *flat* or *level* surface from heel to toe on the sole, not wholly, *but precisely where in this it is hollowed out.* The parts on each side of the level strip would be slightly convex, like the corresponding parts of the foot; not too much so, however, for then the last would be too rounding on the bottom, taking the whole width in view, which is as bad a fault as the hollow, or even worse; as it interferes more with the spreading of the transverse arch, and, by making a *concave* upper surface to the insole of the shoe, compels the ball to tread into just such a hollow as would fit a broken-down, splay foot. The natural inference is that such a shoe would tend to favour the production of just such a foot.

It is believed that the broken-down transverse arch will almost always be found accompanied by the broken-down arch of the instep. Though the latter may exist without the former, yet we suspect that the two incline to go together—that the sinking of the greater arch tends to carry down the other along with it, while a natural weakness of muscle would be a predisposing condition. If there are other causes they are not yet known. The last supposition being correct, then the most direct way to a cure would be to restore the arch of the *instep* to its proper shape and position; which would probably have the same tendency to raise the other, that its depression had to break it down. The grand recipe for this, as already given, is the long heel; which can be made upon any kind of covering, whatever its peculiarities. The use of the muscles of the toes must also come in as an auxiliary help not to be underrated.

Still another remedial measure is the " *righting up* " of the foot. Many, if not most, of the feet that have broken-down arches also tread over inward along the whole side· In such cases the weight of the body, as already stated, falls upon the arch in a wrong direction. The arch, instead of standing *upright* and receiving the weight *directly over* itself, supports the body *while itself leaning over to one side.* Any other kind of arch, in a similar condition, would quickly fall over or settle down; and it is no wonder the foot settles down to a level in the shank. Weak muscles in the ankle and foot of a child will allow the foot to take a one-sided tendency, and it is not impossible the child may inherit something of this weakness from a weak-footed parent, and thus the infirmity be perpetuated. But with the fault existing, however produced, the foot cannot get strong till the arch is restored to its natural perpendicularity. The best manner of righting it up will be described in a chapter farther on. The uprightness will give the muscles a better chance to grow strong, while these assist the operation of the long heel; and possibly it will prove not inferior to either of them in promoting the desired result.

We are sorry that facts from practical effort cannot be given to show a realized success in this direction. But in truth we doubt that an earnest and systematic attempt was ever made to raise up a broken-down foot. All that

can be said is that the methods recommended must necessarily tend toward the restoration of the arch.   But
this alone ought to furnish assurance of success, and encourage an archless-footed person to combine those
methods, and give them a faithful trial.

CHAPTER VI.

IN the last chapter the *instep* was spoken of as a part of the whole arch of the foot. It is now to be looked at from the upper side. When the foot is in its best shape this part is elevated and prominent, with a well-marked and graceful rise from the ball upward, and a distinct projection or convexity at its upward portion, or about half way between the joint and the ankle, which is the upper surface of the first cuneiform bone, or the point where that bone joins the first metatarsal. This place is subject to callosities or thickenings of the skin, resembling corns, but more frequently is affected by soreness without any thickening of the skin. In the broken-down foot there is no convexity here at all, or but very little, the instep being a straight inclined plane from the ankle to the ball, and sometimes even bending downward. Insteps of this kind, whatever bad effects may come from their flatness, are not afflicted in the way just described. Corns and callosities are never known to fasten upon them; an advantage which shows that some good is mixed with evil, in the foot as well as elsewhere. It is the best formed instep, on the contrary, that is most subject to callosity and tenderness.

This tenderness or callosity, whichever it may be, has one cause in the general tightness of the boot worn, and may have two others, arising from the shape of the lasts used. One of these is in the fact that the corresponding part of the last—technically called the *cone* of the instep —does not extend far enough forward, or is shaved off too much—is left *too flat*, for the fitting of well-arched feet. There is not wood enough, proportionally, in the last at this point. The other cause comes from the whole instep, being placed too near the *middle*, instead of on the *side*, where the foot has it. Mr. Watkins, who was referred to in the last chapter, thus explains this defect :

" If the instep is not in the right place, the foot swells in that place. I have seen very troublesome sores on the instep, and very difficult to cure, arising from the misplacing of the instep of the last. By a peculiar measurement* I have been enabled to obviate all difficulty in that

* A measurement for such cases may be taken by drawing the strap-measure from the *point of the instep* around the *heel*, to give the size, while the distance between the same two points, in a straight line, should be taken by the *size-stick*, in the same way we take the *length* of the foot, to show how far forward the point of the instep ought to be located on the last. The measure *around* the foot at the latter place must also be taken.

respect, so that none of my customers now complain of tender insteps. The insteps on ordinary lasts are placed near the middle, which is erroneous, as the point of the instep lies on one side, and not in the centre, and common sense would indicate that the thicker parts of the lasts should be on the side of the large joints and toe, and the thinner on the outside of the foot, where the small toes are placed."

It may seem, at first thought, as we look at a boot after it is made, that the leather will accommodate itself to the shape of the foot with the greatest ease. It appears perfectly pliable, ready to take any form or place that the foot may give to it; and this is true to a great extent, but it is not so entirely. When the boot is made the leather is *stretched*, and worked into a definite shape—that of the last. When a foot large enough to fill it is put inside, if it be of a different form there will be more or less force exerted to change the shape and adapt it to that of the foot. This is one reason of the difficulty often experienced the first time, or first few times, a new boot is worn. The resistance, pressure, and friction may be considerable, or only slight, with a corresponding effect.

This misplacement of the instep is true of the ordinary right-and-left lasts, and it is necessarily still more marked in the *straight* lasts on which the great majority of ladies' boots and shoes are made. If women's insteps do not suffer from this difficulty more than men's, it is because they wear softer material, and boots fitting less tightly than those of men. The latter have an advantage of the former in this respect, as in some others; for while they have right-and-left lasts wholly, with ladies the straight last is the rule, the other the exception. As long as woman does not have her boots and shoes made *right and left*, she is losing one of her "rights," and subjecting her feet to an "oppression" which, unless they can bear a great deal, they will be likely to complain of in an unpleasant way. And this right is not so unimportant, but that it will be found best to give it a little attention, although the remonstrating " subject " may be in a very humble position.

The best thing to be done for feet with sore insteps is to have lasts made to fit them, and their coverings made by some one who knows the real source of the trouble. The sore will generally disappear soon after removing the pressure. The prevention of it is a much better thing, and will come with a more general understanding of the foot's nature, and with the more correctly-shaped lasts and more perfect skilfulness which that knowledge will give to the shoe manufacturer.

There is another deformity of the foot, chiefly of the instep, which might be called the *stub-foot.* It is not the natural short, thick foot of short, stout persons, but seem an unnatural chubbiness, made by prevention of the foot's growth lengthwise. It is an approximation to the Chinese foot—thick and large round the ankle and instep, but short and small at the toes. There is no correct proportion between one part and another. The arch is high, but thick and clumsy, without its natural regularity and beauty. The constant cramping of small shoes, worn when the feet are young, is most probably the cause of such development, by preventing a normal and perfect growth. As the forward parts of the foot, being smaller and weaker, are more easily cramped, the increase of size is at the heel, and around and above the arch.

It is a very Chinese idea of perfection which admires feet of this character. A correctly educated taste prefers to see a foot equally well developed in all its parts, and of a size *proportionate to the size of the whole body*. This is the idea of the artist, as opposed to that of the China-man, and has a reason for it, while the other has none.

If a chance is given the toes to develop themselves before the body gets its full growth, the fault may perhaps be partially outgrown; but after that, the foot will be almost sure to keep the same shape always. The thing to be remedied, is the strange taste which looks upon feet that are abnormally small with any more admiration than would be given to a small head, or short legs, or stumpy fingers. When people who are otherwise intelligent come to see that the foot has the same right to a full and natural growth that belongs to any other part of the body, they will not cramp it with tight boots, or consider a foot of this kind as any more beautiful than a pug nose, a dwarfed limb, or any other lack of development whatever. The defect will then become the result of chance or misfortune only, instead of intention, governed by a false standard of beauty.

It is not, however, intended to deny that there are many
feet which are proportionally too large, made so by some
occupation or habit demanding an extreme development
of bone, muscle, and strength. Nature committed no
mistake in their production. She made them no larger
than was necessary to adapt them to the habits of their
possessor, or of the parents from whom they were inhe-
rited. To attempt to improve them by cramping, is only
to make them worse by distortion. They will probably
decrease their size somewhat in time, if circumstances
favour them in so doing; but if not, they are still no worse
than big hands, big noses, big bodies, or many of those
other unbalanced developments from which none of us
can claim to be entirely free.

Callosities upon the heel, sometimes so bad as to be
called corns, are often troublesome, and mostly so to those
persons whose feet are bony and spare of flesh.   In these,
if they are not broken down, the heel bone, at its upper
part, projects backward distinctly.   If the boot worn slips
at the heel, there is no flesh over the bone to ease the
pressure and friction of the leather, and the skin must
thicken for its own protection. After a while it becomes
so thick, callous, and hard, that every pressure upon it
hurts the bone, as much as before it was formed.   It has
become similar to a hard corn, and must be removed.
This can often be done without any softening, by carefully
cutting, scraping, or lifting up gradually with the knife.
It will probably grow again, and need relifting occa-

sionally as long as the irritation continues. It is due to flat feet to say that they usually escape these annoyances, as well as sores of the instep.

Slipping of the boot at the heel, is almost always the fault of the boot-maker. It may come from bad cutting, from bad fitting of the upper, from bad lasting, and from badly shaped lasts upon which the boots are made. When the cutting is wrong—which affects *men's* boots mainly—it is the leg through the ankle that is too large, or there is some defect that will not allow the upper to *last* properly. Sometimes it is fitted badly, so as to produce the same result. More often than either of these it is the workman, who neglects to draw it over the last in the right way; sometimes from want of knowledge, and sometimes from carelessness or indifference. The error consists in not drawing it over the toe sufficiently tight to make it fit closely at the heel.

A bad fit upon the foot is another cause, in addition to those mentioned; and it is also true that the heels of well-arched feet are more liable to slip than those whose arches are more or less flattened down.

Still another and very decided influence in producing callosities on the heel, is a counter that is hard and stiff at its upper portion. Counters of this kind are very common, and ought to be as commonly avoided. The stiffness of a counter *should be at the bottom of it, where there can hardly be too much, while the upper half, or more, should taper to a thin edge, that is soft and flexible.* Then, while firm at the proper place, it bends and fits snugly to the heel, preventing its slipping ; when, if it stands up straight and stiff throughout, the foot will slip almost invariably.

Lasts, particularly boot lasts, are at fault in this respect generally. Those upon which shoes and slippers are made are so shaped *as to force the shoe to set tightly at the heel and ankle.* The principle upon which they are formed is well known, and is a correct one. It is difficult to see why it should not be carried further in its application, and govern the making of lasts for *boots and gaiters* as well as of those intended for *low shoes.* The necessity is the same in both these styles; there is only a *difference in degree,* which is greater in the *low shoe* and *slipper* than in the *high gaiter* and *boot.* The tightness at the ankle which prevents slipping, is supplied, more or less perfectly, in side spring gaiters, and those that are *laced.* Lacing compels the boot to fit closely, whether it does so easily or not. In men's boots, where there is no lacing, this effect is produced only by having them so small about the heel and ankle that the foot can hardly move at all after it is crowded inside. This may, or may not, be too tight for comfort, but it is doubtful if there is need of its being so for the sake of having a well-fitting boot. The fit can be produced in the same way as in the slipper or shoe, and the demand for doing it is the same, *only not to the same extent.* The slipper has nothing to keep it on the foot, unless strings are resorted to, *except the tightness lengthwise caused by the peculiarity of the last.* A boot, by covering the instep is held more securely, yet it often slips at the heel, and is all the more likely to do so when the foot is well arched.

It seems to us that the way to remedy this trouble in boots is precisely the same as the means taken to *prevent* it in *shoe*s : that is, to make *more spring in the last forward of the instep ; in other words, a greater curve on the bottom.* The amount of this *spring* or curve need not be so great as in the shoe last, for the reason just stated, that the boot is confined at the instep, while the shoe is not, to the same extent. A good shoemaker would not like to make an *Oxford shoe* upon a boot last, although it is laced well up toward the ankle. Why should he be willing to make a boot on it, when the boot is confined at the instep no more than the shoe? There is the same danger of slipping in both cases, and why should it not be guarded against in the same way? Every one who has made or sold shoes knows that a slipper, or low shoe of any kind, will fit on the foot much better if made on a shoe last; that it is less liable to be loose at the sides, and to show big wrinkles across the ball; that, in short, it *must* be made on such a last. The same reasoning and the same rule applies almost as well to the boot or gaiter. If there is any exception, it is the side-spring boot, with its elastic sides to draw the surface smooth, and even this is not an exception when the material is leather, though it may be when cloth of any kind is used. In fact, there is no kind of foot clothing manufactured but would have a better fit upon the foot, both in front and at the heel, sides, and ankle, if a last more closely resembling the common shoe or slipper last was used in the making. There may not be, and we are confident there *is* not, a necessity for having it so *flat in the shank* as the common slipper last, nor so *wide* through the same region, but the upward curve of the forward part should be nearly or quite as great. The curve of the shank might be very nearly the same as that of the hollow of the foot, while at the toes it may curve, we will say, one-half as much as the whole bend of the toes in walking. This form makes it a shoe last at the fore part, while the shank is but little different from the ordinary *boot* last. The part between the heel and instep need not be so wide at the bottom, nor, perhaps, so narrow at the top, as the best shaped lasts for shoes. It is believed possible, however, to make the shank sufficiently wide, at a slight distance *above* the bottom, to accommodate the foot easily, while it may be suddenly narrowed *below* sufficiently to allow a narrow-shanked sole to be made upon it, if desired, without difficulty. If so, this would be the blending of *taste* with *comfort* in the fit. The outside edge would be a little *lower* than the other, as it is in the foot. Perhaps the whole may be well described as half-way between the extremes of the two different styles. There would be no difference between those designed for men and those for women, except in width and bulk—none in the general form.

It may be feared that a tongued boot—patent leather or Napoleon—may be more difficult to draw on the foot if made upon a last of this style. We believe that it can make but very little difference, probably not any after the boot is bent in the shank, while it *will* do much to prevent slipping at the heel when cut with a large ankle, as is usually the case. The pitch of the leg will be very nearly the same when on the last as when the boot is worn.

It may be observed, however, that an improvement has lately been made in many lasts by giving them a greater degree of this curve on the bottom. But it is easy to carry it to an extreme. The sole can be curved too much as well as left too straight. Men's lasts of medium size have been made with the toes raised an inch and a half above the level of the ball and heel; which is half an inch more than is necessary, or useful. Too much spring, in a thick-soled, stiff boot, prevents the straightening of the toes, while in a thin one, where the toes can be straightened, it may create longitudinal wrinkles in the upper, near the sole at the inside joint. An average spring of an inch in men's lasts, and three-fourths of an inch in those for women, is not far from the proper standard.

Forms of lasts have always been subject to change. Fifteen or twenty years ago boot lasts were made very hollow in the shank, and very much curved upward at the toe. After that came the stub-toes—flat in shank, and

7

with scarcely any curve at all ; and, in addition to all the changes fashion has imposed, besides the two indicated, every manufacturer seems to have 'a style of his own, more or less distinct. The principles which should govern their form seem to be very loosely understood, and hence all the differing shapes and styles.

All this is exactly the opposite of what it should be. We have no more right to change the shape of lasts every few years than we have to change that of the foot, and to do this, for it amounts to nothing less, when Nature has formed it exactly in the best way to adapt it to its design and use, is simple absurdity. To change either is just as foolish as it would be to make hats that would flatten the head on the back or sides, and compel it to grow in an upward direction. The whole matter of the shape of lasts is something which fashion has no right to meddle with, unless, it may be, to round or square the toes. It has no right to *narrow* them beyond a certain limit, nor even at all except from the outside. The business of the last-maker is to learn what is the true shape of the natural, healthy foot, and then to imitate it as closely as possible, making only the slight differences for different kinds of coverings that have been pointed out. And when so formed, let it be considered as a thing not to be altered, except to make it resemble the foot still more perfectly. Fashion and taste may change and dictate the cut and style of the upper parts of the boot or shoe to almost any extent, but they must not be allowed to shorten the length of the heel, nor to interfere in any manner with the shape of the last.

We have been somewhat particular in description, for the sake of influencing the makers of lasts and boots, as well as for the comfort of those who are to wear the latter. When these principles govern in its manufacture, the boot will fit almost as easily at the first putting on as it will after a week's wearing. The trouble of "breaking in" will be nearly abolished. It may also be promised that slipping at the heel will be of rare occurrence, and the callosities produced by it be got rid of with little difficulty. When once removed they will not be likely to come again, with a boot that causes no irritation.

CHAPTER VII.

Inclinations of the Feet—How to Make them Tread Squarely—Peculiar Lasts—Weak Ankles—Cultivation of Muscle—Turning in of the Toes.

THERE remains still one other defect to be noticed—· that of treading upon the side of the foot. This is a very common fault, and seems to be a habit often acquired quite early. The feet appear to leave the old, upright way of getting through the world, and take a sidewise deviation. Having commenced losing their uprightness when young, they, unless speedily helped, seldom recover it entirely afterward. The individual who possesses such unfortunate *inclinations* never has the satisfaction of knowing what it is to stand up in *perfect rectitude.* Whether the physical leaning of the feet has any tendency to create a moral one-sidedness may be considered an open question. It is hardly safe to say that it does *not*, when we know that the whole carriage, attitude, and dress of the individual has an effect upon the condition of the mind. But leaving that to be settled as it may, we must see what can be done to straighten the feet up to their natural position.

Feet that tread upon the *inside* are, many of them, *flattened* somewhat at the same time. This latter fault may come from any of the influences previously pointed out, or from a natural weakness of the muscles and ligaments of the ankle, which condition frequently exists in children. When this is the case, the arch of the foot being turned, the weight of the body is improperly directed upon it—that is, the arch bears this weight slightly upon one side instead of directly *over* itself. This tends to break it down and make the foot flat. The flatness, if already existing, may tend to throw the foot still more toward the side. Either way, the first thing to be done is to counteract the flatness by a sufficiently long heel under the shoe, to support the arch. The shoe should also be made upon a flat-bottomed last, and one that will compel it to draw tight along the sides and ankle. Another requisite is that the counter shall be very *stiff* on the inside, while on the opposite side it should be *weak*. It should also be high as well as firm, sometimes *very* high, as when the ankle requires very much support. When, however, it reaches so high as to touch the prominences of the joint, it must be carefully thinned on the edge to prevent chafing the bone. If the weakness is but slight, the principal part of the stiffness may be near the bottom, where a good deal of it will do no harm.

All persons having feet thus turned should patronize

the last maker before expecting to accomplish much toward correcting them. An ordinary last is, in these
cases, good for nothing. It needs to be straight, or nearly
so, on its outside edge, from heel to ball, and that part
between the heel and instep—the back half of it—should
be very full on the outside, while it should be much hollowed out on the *inside.* In other words without altering
the general form of the front part, *the bulk of the wood in
the back and middle parts should incline toward, and be
on, the outside.* The bottom of the last, *particularly at
the heel,* may then be thinned off at the outside edge of
the *sole,* leaving it deepest, or thickest, relatively, at its
inside. It then has the appearance of being *inclined over
outwardly.* The shoe or boot made upon it would really
be inclined outwardly, and possess a tendency to push the
foot which wore it over in the same direction. This is its
precise intention. The maker must not forget to see that
the upper is lasted over equally on both sides, or more on
the outside, if either. Then it is just such a shoe as
would fit easily and comfortably a foot that treads outside ; and *for that very reason* it is exactly such a one as
ought to be worn by a foot that treads *inwardly.* All the
force exerted by the stiffness of the counter, and the *inclination of the whole shoe,* goes toward righting up the foot
and pushing it over outwardly. Still there is nothing that
can *hurt* the foot—only a steady and gentle pressure in
the right direction, which does not interfere with the use
of the muscles.

In extreme cases a further precaution may be taken by building the heels more upon the inside than the other, and raising them a little the highest on that side, fortifying them still more by some large nails, while the *outside* is not guarded at all. The inside edge of the sole, if sufficiently thick, may be treated in the same way.

We have said the last should be *flat*. It ought to be quite as much so as the foot ; and the long heel must not be forgotten. Of course if there is *no* flatness of the shank, as is sometimes the case, there need be none in the last.

This plan of treatment will not only right up the foot, but we believe it will be a great help toward raising the flattened arch. At least, it ought not to be neglected in any case of flat-foot associated with treading inward ; for as long as the foot treads on the inside, there is one cause— weight wrongly directed on the arch—constantly operating to break it down. And this might defeat all the efforts for its restoration.

Those feet that tread *outside* need exactly the same treatment recommended for the others, only, in the shoes made for them, it must be directed in a way exactly opposite. The stiffness of the counter must be on the outside, as also the guarding of the heel. The last must be straight and *very full* upon the *inside*. The main bulk of the wood between the heel and instep should be on that side, projecting well over the bottom at the ball, while it is spare, thinned, or hollowed on the other. The bottom should be thinned off at the inner edge, so that when placed upon a level surface it seems to lean that way. In a word, it will look as though it would fit beautifully a foot that treads *inward. Then it is just adapted for one that goes outward.* The whole shape and fit of a boot made upon such a last exerts an easy pressure, tending to right up the foot and force it to tread on the opposite side. The principle has not heretofore been generally recognized. Let it not be forgotten that the last that would appear to fit a foot that treads outward is just the one to be used for a foot that goes inward, and *vice versa.* When this is acted upon, the principal step is taken in overcoming the difficulty.

But as many persons having such feet preserve the natural form of them by treading the boots outside, it is about as well to let them go so, as attempt to right them up, even if a little more leather is thus worn out. On the contrary, when the tendency is to tread *inside*, the remedy can not be applied too soon if it is wished to avoid the big joints that result from such a habit.

Without the lasts here mentioned, however, a little temporary improvement can still be effected in those feet that tread over but slightly, by what shoemakers call "working under" the sole of the shoe on the side opposite that which treads over, and by also putting a piece of leather on the last *above the sole or bottom*, to make room in the upper at that side without increasing the width of the sole. The *sole* may be "worked full" on the *treading-over* side at the same time.

Feet that tread outside generally, if not always, have good arches.

The directions here given, if put in practice by a shoe-maker who can appreciate and apply them thoroughly, will, it is believed, straighten up and cure any case of treading-over feet that can be helped at all. And this probably includes the majority of instances. The adoption of such lasts has never been fairly tried, as far as we know, and we are quite confident they will prove successful.

The turning over of the foot is believed to be sometimes occasioned in children by their being obliged or encouraged to stand or walk upon them for too long a time, when making their first attempts, in infancy. The bones, ligaments, and muscles being all soft, tender, and weak at this period, they may be forced into almost any shape by pressure or overstraining. This is something worthy of careful attention from parents. It is very easy to let a child contract a habit of walking which will render the feet and legs deformed through a whole lifetime. It is also very easy to prevent it, and give the child a natural, upright, easy, and graceful walk by taking a little pains at the proper period. And it should also be remembered that crooked feet and ankles are more easily straightened while they are young than when the foot has obtained its growth, and every part become firmly settled in its false position.

The legs and feet may turn inward, developing knock-knees and flat-foot, or outward, growing into bow-legs, with the feet invariably treading over the opposite way. If a child grows up with either of these distortions, after being born with sound limbs, which might have been continued in their natural perfection, there is, on the part of somebody, a sad lack of duty.

It is quite possible, also, that this habit may be adopted by children sometimes from wearing a shoe that hurts the foot. The sufferer may turn it on one side to avoid a peg, or some rough projection on the insole, and in this way the fault may be developed in some of those cases where one foot treads over, while the other stands upright. And children will often get into an awkward manner of standing or walking, even without any reason for it—from sheer carelessness—and require a great deal of watching, in order to train up their feet correctly.*

It is to be borne in mind that in all cases of weak ankles, except those incurably so, the object should be to support them no more than is necessary ; but instead, to allow the muscles to be used as much as possible for the sake of *strengthening them.* When the whole support comes from

---

* Another reason for care in guarding against weak ankles is thus given in a work upon the "Theory and Practice of the Movement-Cure," by Dr. Charles F. Taylor.

"Weak ankles, often the result of the ungraceful, and, in other respects, pernicious fashion of wearing high, narrow-heeled shoes, straining them by their rolling about, etc., may be the exciting cause of *lateral curvature of the spine.* The weaker ankle is generally the *left,* and the individual soon forms the habit of standing on the right foot. The lower portion of the spine is thrown to the *left,* and the dorsal portion necessarily thrown to the *right.*" In another place he repeats : "We find that almost without exception, in curvature to the *right,* the *left* ankle is much weaker than the other. Movements of the foot must be employed, such as inward and outward flexion, twisting the whole leg from the hip, and many others, calculated to strengthen the left leg, hip, and ankle."

braces—in the shoe or outside of it—there is nothing left
to be done by the muscles on the side of the foot and leg,
and consequently they remain weak. The law of growth
and strength is use, exercise, or labour. Hence, though
guards and braces are sometimes required for weak-ankled
children, there ought to be plenty of room between them
and the foot ; and it will be well to discard them as soon
as a leather stiffening in the shoe can be safely substituted.

There are many movements of the *Light Gymnastics* that
for weak ankles would be highly beneficial. It would be
well, where there is an opportunity, to adopt all those movements in which the muscles of the feet are called into play
such as charging, leaning, bracing, springing on the toes,
and, in short, almost the whole routine of exercises ; and
to practice them, cautiously at first, but thoroughly, until
the muscles and ligaments become strong enough to do
their duty in bracing up the foot without any assistance.

There are many feet in which the *toes* turn inward in
walking—a habit which may be easily corrected by a little
care and perseverance, and the subject of it enabled to
go on his way rejoicing in the knowledge that he has
gained a respectable walk in place of one that was ridiculously awkward. All that is required to change the habit
is to develope the strength of the muscles by calling them
into exercise. An every-day practice of turning the feet
outward as far as possible, for a few minutes at a time,
will do a great deal. If, in addition to this, the step is
constantly watched, the toes being kept turned out until

the muscles are tired, and then, after resting by a return to the old step, the toes are again forced outward, and this is repeated continuously for a few weeks, the awkwardness will be entirely gone. The practice of light gymnastics is a good corrective for this fault; and the dancing-school is another equally excellent. It is to be hoped that both of them will have their due influence in this respect, till an ungraceful walk is far less common than it is now. With such easy means of correcting and avoiding these faults, any one who will not make a little effort for that purpose, deserves, to say the least, a good share of ridicule.*

There is a less number of feet that are turned *too much* outward, and these can be brought into their right place by the same means directed in the opposite way. The only trouble with them usually is a habit, or a weakness of particular muscles. If the toes are turned in, and perseveringly kept so for a short time, a great difference will be discovered. A further continuance in well-doing will bring its reward in an easy, natural, and graceful step.

* As a matter not wholly out of place, it may be said that the graceful walker stands upright, and in taking a step uses the muscles and joints of the *hip*, the *knee*, and the *toes*. Many people use the toes but very little, and their step lacks *spring, elasticity, life,* and *grace;* while others do not use the muscles in front of the hip enough, and their walk has no dignity. Instead of swinging the whole leg, they seem as though kicking their feet along ahead of them, swinging only that half of it ¡below the knee. Stiff covering on the feet, or very high heels under them, effectually prevent all gracefulness in walking.

Those feet that are wholly turned, or deformed by being drawn up at the heel or toe, and those impaired by disease of the structure, are cases belonging to the surgeon and physician. Many of them might probably have been prevented by calling in the surgeon's aid during the childhood of the unfortunate possessor. Let us hope that few who can be saved from such disfigurement will be allowed to suffer from it through ignorance or culpable negligence in the future.

CHAPTER VIII.

Corns, Bunions, and Callosities—How they Originate—Nature of
the Skin—Various Causes of Corns—How to Remove Them—
Quotations from the Medical Books—Nature and Treatment of
Bunions.

WE come now to another class of difficulties to which
the foot is subject, though they affect the outside
mainly, not its structure, and which appropriately call for
a notice here, and for some hints concerning their nature
and treatment. Almost every one, at some period in a
lifetime, forms their unpleasant acquaintance; and to
know how to avoid them entirely, or to destroy and remove
them at pleasure, may be considered information worth
possessing. Although we lack the familiar practical
knowledge of the man who makes corns his profession,
the reader shall have the benefit of as much as we are
able to supply.

A common corn is caused by friction or irritation of the
skin—the chafing and pressure of the foot against the
leather of the boot, or the crowding of the toes against
each other. The skin thickens and hardens to protect

itself in the same way that it does upon the hands or other parts of the body exposed to rough contact, the fact and law of which are familiar to everybody. As the irritation is continued the skin continues growing harder and thicker, until a large and ugly corn is produced. To understand its nature more fully, and why it assumes a sharp point, thus turning its protection into a torture, it will be necessary to explain something more of the nature of the skin itself.

There are two layers of membrane composing the skin —the *cutis vera*, dermis, or true skin, which is the inner portion; and the cuticle, epidermis, or scarf-skin, which is the outside layer. The dermis, or true skin, consists mainly of a net-work or web of fibrous material, having outside of this a net-work of capillary blood-vessels and lymphatics, interwoven with still another net-work, of nerves, both blood-vessels and nerves terminating in projecting or upright loops, each loop formed of a blood-vessel and a nerve-cord, the two being together side by side. These loops, which are the most extremely sensitive portion of the skin, are called *papillæ*, and they form the projecting fine ridges that are seen on the palm of the hand, where their abundance gives the hand its superior sense of feeling or touch. All these parts—the fibrous meshes, the blood-vessels, nerves, and loops of papillæ— are microscopically minute.

The outside skin or cuticle has no blood-vessels or

nerves, and hence no life or sensation, but seems to be a *covering* to protect the true skin, and to modify or diminish its otherwise too extreme sensitiveness; besides being of use in other ways to the general system. It is that part which is raised up when a blister is produced; and the sensitiveness of the papillæ under it, where it is taken off, shows its necessity. The matter of which it is formed is secreted or poured out by the true skin, and is the same matter which, when dried and hardened in various degrees, becomes the thick skin on the sole of the foot, the callous place on the hand or elsewhere, the dandruff of the head, the hair on any part of the body, the nails of fingers and toes, the hard portion of warts, and the hard or soft corn. All these are essentially the same thing under different modifications. It is constantly worn off from the external surface, and as constantly added to at the under side.

This internal or under-side layer of the cuticle is commonly distinguished as the *rete mucosum,* and contains a colouring matter secreted from the true skin, which, as it is greater or less in quantity gives the different shades of complexion; the semi-transparent nature of the matter outside allowing it to show through. The oil tubes and perspiratory ducts take their rise immediately under the skin, and find their way to the surface, while nerves and blood-vessels traverse it forth and back.

Some further idea of the nature of the skin may be gained by observing a piece of thick sole-leather in which that part called the grain is the cuticle or epidermis, and the thicker portion is the dermis, or *cutis vera.*

Now, when any portion of these sensitive loops is injuriously irritated by pressure or friction, they sometimes push entirely through the cuticle, growing large and covering themselves with hard cuticular matter, thus forming the warts that appear on the hands and other parts of the body. Some corns, we believe, are produced in a similar way—a larger number of the papillæ projecting and being covered completely and thickly with epidermis, which, becoming dry and hard, still further pains the sore and sensitive papillæ as it is pressed upon by the boot. This kind of corn can be cured only as a wart is removed—by burning the papillæ, or, as they are called in the wart, the *roots;* thus changing the structure of the skin, or, in other words, making a scar.

Ordinarily a hard corn commences at a point, or by the irritation of a small surface of the skin, or only a *few* of the papillæ. From this point an increased supply of the cuticular matter is pushed out in every direction to protect them, growing harder as the process advances, and being more pressed against by the shoe, while the increasing external pressure incites the foot to push out a still larger corn. Thus it grows ; and as the matter first thrown out is the first to become hardened, a point is formed, and the pressure forces it into the flesh, which is compelled to retire before it. The longer this is continued the larger the surface of skin that is made sore, the larger and more

8

conical in shape the corn becomes, and the farther its point is forced into the flesh.

This description is more especially true of the smaller corns; those which extend over a large surface being, probably, originated by a slighter irritation of a larger portion of the skin; hence they have less of a point and penetrate less deeply.

Soft corns appear between the toes, and are soft for the reason that, so situated, they are kept moist by perspiration. Some of them are secretions of epidermis having no centre or point, but thrown out from the foot at the bottom and sides of the space between the toes, and giving a sensation as of some foreign body, like a pea or a gravel stone, confined there. There may be others that are accompanied by projections of the papillæ.

It is to be noticed that a corn is thus composed wholly of cuticular matter, and is entirely outside of the true skin.

It has been suggested that here is an instance in which the remedial effort made by Nature converts itself into a diseased and painful action, defeating its primary purpose and creating a worse condition than the one sought to be relieved. But this is not correct. Nature does not put the boot on the foot, nor continue its wear after the corn has originated. On the contrary, if her intimations were heeded, the boot would be discarded the first time it pinched, and there is every reason to believe that then the growth of the corn would be discontinued, and what had already formed would disappear. It is stated in medical works that persons confined by sickness for a considerable time have had their corns entirely leave them without any treatment at all, simply because there was no pressure to keep up the irritation, and conse-. quently no demand for their existence.

It has been generally considered that tight boots were the great *cause* of all the corns and bunions with which the feet have been tormented, and tight boots have accordingly been cursed from toe to heel for their mischiev-.ous qualities in this respect. Though it is true that the unnecessary tightness of boots is a principal source of corns, there are others that may not be overlooked. *Loose* boots, that allow the heel to slip up and down, or the whole foot to slide forward at every step, are effective in the production of these annoyances. Hard, stiff leather is another quite efficient thing in this way. Whether the boot be tight or loose makes not much difference, if it be stiff and hard. Large wrinkles over the joint may sometimes have an effect of the same kind, especially if the leather is no softer "than it ought to be." High heels, that pitch the foot forward, and keep it constantly bearing against the leather over the toes, have a great tendency to develop corns. The drawing together of the toes by boots and shoes that are *narrow* at this point, forcing the toes to crowd against each other, and pushing out the great-toe joint, is one of the most productive of all causes. When occurring upon the bottom of the foot, a peg or some hard projection of the insole of the boot is the agent to which they may be attributed. Between the toes they are most frequently developed, probably by the pressure of a boot that is too narrow, not only at the ends of the toes, but at their roots or metatarsal joints.

Bunions, we believe, are never found except upon the joint of the great toe, and the projection of this joint, from the wearing of short and narrow-toed shoes, can not be otherwise than strongly influential in producing them. From wearing foot-coverings of this fashion, which is almost the only kind we have at present, there is the constant tendency of the joint to enlarge, widen, and project. This increases its pressure against the leather, and may even create a pressure where there was none at the time the boot was first worn. It is not strange, therefore, that bunions make their appearance under such circumstances.

Thus it is seen that, setting aside the habit of wearing boots that are tight enough to pinch the foot, there is already found an abundant cause for corns. It ought to be sufficiently obvious that the principal characteristics of the present foot-covering—the narrow toes, being often short besides, and the high heels—are corn-producing in all their tendencies. If to these is added the practice, as with many persons, of wearing boots and shoes that are too tight for comfort, and often too narrow on the sole, there is ample reason for the fact that corned feet are numerous.

We do not know what first induced people to wear boots

unnecessarily tight, unless it was the Chinese idea of taste, which desired to prevent the full development of the feet, or make them appear as small as possible. If this be still the motive, it is only necessary to repeat that a true taste demands that a foot be of a size proportionate to the size of the whole body, whether that be large or small. If it is to make the boot fit more smoothly and handsomely, then the object is more often defeated than accomplished. A boot that is too tight—tight enough to be uncomfortable— is not the boot that best fits the foot. It will have as many wrinkles in it as a loose one, and even more, if the leather be thin, while the foot can not go into it naturally. The best fitting boot or shoe is one made of the right shape to adapt it to the particular foot ; which is just snug enough to confine it without any uneasy feeling ; and into which it goes easily and naturally to its proper position. There is sufficient length to allow the toe to move without pressure on the nail, and sufficient width to let the toes lie side by side, in which position they appear much better than when piled one over another. There are no wrinkles made by loose leather—none by over-tightness. The room is entirely filled, while at the same time the foot is easy, and can make its natural movements in walking with ease and grace ; which it can not do when squeezed into a boot that is too tight. A person wearing a tight boot has a stiff and unnatural walk, which can not be compensated by any beauty of the fit so gained, provided it *is* gained. There are only the soft and fleshy feet that can bear compression with any benefit to their appearance, and with these still the same rule is equally good—they must not be squeezed more than comfort will allow. If complaint is made that the upper leather stretches out, and the foot treads over the sole, and spreads and sprawls about more than appears neat and proper, it is only to be replied that if a shoe of the right shape, and sufficiently wide is worn, there will be no trouble of this kind.

On the whole, tight-boot-wearing is a humbug. It is entirely unnecessary, doing no good, while often defeating itself when its object is to improve the foot's appearance. Besides the ordinary discomfort created by it, the whole tendency of extreme tightness is toward corns and deformity.

How much, now, it may be inquired, is meant by *extreme tightness ?* The answer is—*discomfort.* A new boot or shoe that fits as it should, may be worn without serious discomfort for several hours, or half a day, when first put on. After three or four days it may be worn all the time. It ought not to be expected that it can be worn constantly at first ; for if loose enough, for this it will soon be too loose for a handsome fit. Then, an article that is tight for a foot belonging to a weak and delicate organization, with a feeble circulation of blood, may be perfectly easy to a foot of the same size and shape belonging to a strong, healthy constitution with an energetic circulation ; and for the same reason a person can wear a tighter shoe when young than when advanced in life, or failing in health ; but either of these, and at any time, may be governed by the rule, that positive discomfort indicates extreme tightness. There are some kinds of material that stretch considerably under the foot's pressure, and boots made from these should be a little tighter at first than those made of firmer stock. Besides, there are some feet so sensitive that very slight pressure or friction will develope corns on them, and such must wear a softer material than is worn by feet that are more hardy. The question of tightness is somewhat complicated by such considerations. Most of us, however, can usually tell for ourselves what is tight, and we have no right to decide for others.

Ordinary hard corns, when young, may be removed by scraping up the callous skin around the borders and prying out carefully with a pocket knife. There is no need of cutting through the under skin. In more difficult cases some further treatment will be necessary, and for them we quote the following methods, the first from Cooper's "Dictionary of Surgery."

"Wide, soft shoes should be worn. Such means are not only requisite for a radical cure, but they alone often effect it. Though the radical cure is thus easy, few obtain it, because their perseverance ceases, as soon as they experience the wished-for relief.

"When business or other circumstances prevent the patient from adopting this plan, and oblige him to stand or walk a good deal, still it is possible to remove all

pressure from the corn. For this purpose from eight to·
twelve pieces of linen, smeared with an emollient ointment,.
and having an aperture cut in the middle exactly adapted
to the corn, are to be laid over each other, and so applied
to the foot that the corn is to lie in the opening in such a
manner that it can not be touched by the shoe or stocking.-
When the plaster has been applied some weeks the corn
commonly disappears without other means. Should the·
corn be on the sole of the foot, it is only necessary to·
put in the shoe a *felt* sole wherein a whole has been cut,
corresponding to the situation, size, and figure of the in-·
duration.

"A corn may also be certainly, permanently, and speedily
eradicated by the following method, especially when the·
plaster and felt with a hole in it are employed at the same
time. · The corn is to be rubbed twice a day with an emollient ointment, such as that of marshmallows, or with the·
volatile liniment, which is still better; and in the interim it is.
to be covered with a softening plaster. Every morning and
evening the foot is to be put, for half an hour, in warm.
water, and while there the corn is to be well rubbed with
soap. Afterwards all the soft, white, pulpy matter outside·
of the corn is to be scraped off with a blunt knife; but the
scraping must be left off the moment the patient begins to·
complain of pain from it. The same treatment is to be
persisted in without interruption until the corn is totally
extirpated, which is generally effected in eight or twelve·
days. If left off sooner the corn grows again."

The "Hydropathic Enclyclopædia" recommends a more summary mode of dealing.

"These well-known toe-tormenters are produced by light shoes or boots. The first principle of cure is to give the feet a respectable 'area of freedom;' and the second is, to soak them in warm water and shave off the horny substance, and then touch them with the nitric or nitro-muriatic acid. When the corn is inflamed or highly irritable, the tepid foot-bath should be employed to remove this condition before the acid is applied. The *aqua-regia*—nitro-muriatic acid—is the ordinary secret remedy of the 'corn-curers.' When the corn is fully formed, or ripe, a membrane separates it from the true skin, so that it can be taken off without injuring that surface; and this circumstance enables professional chiropodists to 'elevate the grain' on the point of a penknife, after an application of the acid."

Another mode, similar in character, is taken from a late work by Dr. Ira Warren.

"Corns should be shaved down close, after being soaked in warm water and soap, and then covered with a piece of wash-leather or buck-skin, on which lead plaster is spread, a hole being cut in the leather the size of the corn. They may be softened so as to be easily scooped out by rubbing glycerine on them. Manganic acid destroys warts and corns rapidly."

Still another, and one very easy to practice, is from Dr. Calvin Cutter's "Anatomy, Physiology, and Hygiene."

"To remove these painful excrescences, take a thick

piece of soft leather, somewhat larger than the corn; in the centre punch a hole of the size of the summit of the corn; spread the leather with adhesive plaster, and apply it around the corn. The hole in the leather may be filled with a paste made of soda and soap on going to bed. In the morning remove it, and wash with warm water. Repeat this for several successive nights, and the corn will be removed. The only precaution is, not to repeat the application so as to cause pain."

It is altogether probable that the last treatment here advised for hard corns would be equally effective for soft ones, if we could contrive to cover up the surrounding parts with a plaster so as to admit of its application. The other remedies are, to keep continually cutting away at them with the knife, or burn them out thoroughly with caustic.

In all these cures the essential parts of the treatment are, first, the emollient ointment or warm water to soften the skin and remove soreness; then caustics—soap and soda, nitric, muriatic, and manganic acids—to destroy the mass of the corn; after which the remainder is lifted out with a knife; the leather and felt serving as a protection from the shoe.

It is said, and with considerable evidence to support the statement, that ordinary mild corns may be cured in a couple of weeks by winding a cotton rag around the toe or foot, so as to cover the corn with several thicknesses, and then keeping this bandage constantly wet by bathing the feet twice a day in cold water. To which it may be added, that many corns will probably disappear if constantly kept moist and soft in any manner, provided the external irritation is entirely removed.

Very often it is the case that new corns, both hard and soft, grow up in the places where they have been taken away before, re-appearing, some of them, several times; and it is a question if the common practice of putting leather with a hole in it around the corn does not tend to make the latter grow up again by pressing on the edges of the cavity. It is perhaps better, therefore, that the leather or felt be worn for some time after the corn is gone, to keep the pressure of the boot away from the part till it has regained its natural condition, and it is well to make the hole in the plaster *so large*, that even the border of the sensitive cavity will not be touched. When a surface has been secreting corn-material for a length of time, it is not strange that it should continue the habit without much provocation. In these cases where the corn grows again, it may perhaps be advisable to touch the most central part, or place of the *point*, with nitric acid or some other caustic, to destroy the papillæ, and change the structure of the skin, as is done with a wart; where it is so effectual that the wart never re-appears. It is not necessary to burn the surrounding surface, or make anything more than a very small burn anywhere. The acid should be applied with some sharp-pointed instrument, just wet with it, so there shall be no danger of putting on too much. If there is any fear of creating too much inflammation, it can be postponed till the acute sensitiveness has become somewhat abated.

For soft corns it is doubtful whether any other treatment than burning will be completely successful, though it may be well to try some other method first. Burning is rather severe, but reasonably sure, and a thousand times better, than to suffer from the corn. But little acid need be applied at a time, and as soon as the under skin becomes inflamed the desired effect is accomplished; for when it heals, the corn is "done for" and gone. Something soft may be put between the toes to separate them, and prevent any unnecessary irritation during the process.

Corns on the bottom of the foot are amenable to caustic like the rest, the felt sole with a hole in it being used for protection during the operation.

Inflamed and suppurated corns are to be cut down as much as possible and lanced, according to Erichsen—one of the best authorities—though it would seem to one unacquainted with the matter that they might be removed like the others. They are intensely painful, and a surgeon's skill is necessary to treat them properly.

Some of the medical books represent that there is more or less danger in using caustics in severe cases, where the patient is an old person, or one of feeble vitality, or extreme nervous sensibility. It is always well to proceed safely, and have medical advice before operating on such a patient.

In addition to the ordinary hard and soft varieties, *black* and *bleeding* corns are described by one writer on the subject, some of which are reported very difficult to cure and dangerous to manage ; their injudicious removal being liable to result in convulsions, and even lockjaw and death ; all of which frightful consequences may be accepted as inducements to avoid the productive first causes of the trouble.

In regard to the treatment of *bunions*, the following from the " Hydropathic Encyclopædia," is the only thing we are able to find in the books.

" This affliction, though generally regarded as a kind of corn, is really an inflammation and swelling of the *bursa mucosa*,* at the inside of the ball of the great toe ; it often produces a distortion of the metatarsal joint of the great toe, and is produced by the same causes as corns. The treatment is, warm foot-baths when the part is very tender and irritable ; at other times frequent cold baths ; and when a horny substance, resembling a corn, appears externally, the application of caustic. I have known bad corns and bunions cease to be troublesome after the patient had been a few months under hydropathic treatment for other complaints."

The straightening of the great toe in the manner previously described will probably do more toward the relief and cure of bunions than any other remedy. The ma-

* The *bursa mucosa* is a synovial membrane lining the joint, and secreting a lubricating fluid, like similar membranes in other joints.

terial of a shoe for that purpose should, of course, be soft
—the softest kinds of calfskin are good—but not of *too*
yielding a nature, or the toe and joint will force it into
their own abnormal shape in spite of the form of the shoe,
unless this can be prevented by a stiffening piece of sole-
leather at the ball (see Chapter Four), because the parts
tend to assume their old position, and do so, as far as the
leather will allow. With the ordinary shoe, all that can
be done, is to give the foot the softest of leather—buck-
skin, when obtainable, is the best—and make the shoe
over a last having also a big joint upon it, made of sole-
leather, in the exact place to fit that of the foot, and thus
allow it plenty of room.

The callosities that come upon the heel, instep, or other
part of the foot, can almost always be lifted or scraped off,
without the necessity of using caustic, and there is less
probability of their re-appearing after the cause is removed
than in the case of corns. But if the pressure that caused
them first is continued, of course they grow again. When
they are so bad as to make it difficult to remove them
without softening, they can be subjected to the same treatment which softens corns.

Sore insteps, big joints, and corns, when no positive
means are adopted for their cure or removal, may often
be made tolerably comfortable by having the shoe carefully adapted to fit them. This is done by making leather
corns or joints on the lasts before the shoes are made.

Particular places in a shoe can also, generally, be stretched, so as to render them much more easy.*

Trusting that those readers who are not able to avail themselves of the services of a professional chiropodist, will here find a sufficient guide for the management of ordinary difficulties of this kind, attention will next be called to a re-statement of some of the ideas and points of argument previously advanced in this treatise.

* It will, perhaps, not be amiss here to give a cure for *chilblains*, taken from a recent work upon the "Movement Cure," by Dr. George H. Taylor. It consists in raising the foot, with the shoe upon it, and giving it thirty or forty smart blows upon the sole with a heavy stick of convenient length to be handled. The shock upon the foot dissipates the congestion of blood in the capillary vessels under the skin, which causes the intense itching and smart. It is so simple that every one afflicted ought to try it, and is asserted to be, with few repetitions, a permanent cure.

CHAPTER IX.

Recapitulation—Lasts for Individual Feet—Possibility of all Fee
being Well Fitted in their Clothing—Ease and Grace of Movement—A Last Word for Children.

WE have heretofore endeavoured to show what is the
true, normal shape of the healthy foot, as recognized by science, art, and common sense ; that in it the
toes lie directly forward of the metatarsal bones, in the
same line, having plenty of room for all of them to come
to the ground, or the surface on which they tread ; that
there is no occasion for grown-in-nails, big joints, or corns
until after the adoption of false habits in the manner of
the foot's clothing ; that the elevation of the instep is
made by a well-formed and distinct arch, the breaking-
down of which, as manifested in the flattened instep and
elongated heel, is unnatural ; that all the various deformities, weaknesses, and ailments pointed out and remarked
upon are so many vitiations or perversions of the foot's
condition. It has been made plain, also, *that all our
present habits and ways of dressing the feet tend, more or
less directly and strongly, toward this depravity and distortion.* We have seen that the common sole, by being

curved where it should be straight—on its inside line—inevitably draws the great toe to one side, and all the toes too closely together, pushing out the joint, creating corns between and outside the toes, and lameness or bunion at the joint itself; that this tendency is *increased* by *straight* and *narrow-toed* soles; that it is made still worse by *high heels*, which pitch the foot far forward; while the practice of wearing boots and shoes that are too short makes yet another addition toward the production of the whole bad result.

So also it is seen that the old-fashioned *short heels*, so long worn, have had an influence in producing the broken-down arch of the flat-foot; while other defects in the construction of the foot's covering manifest themselves by callosities on the heel and instep, the turning over to one side, and the pressure, squeezing, and general discomfort in the fit.

We have, still further, tried to indicate what is the true, natural, and proper shape of *last*, and wherein it differs from those in common use. This it will do no harm to re-state. First it was proven that a correctly-formed last was not a thing to be changed by fashion or custom, but on the contrary, to be as permanent in its form as that of the foot which it imitates; that one of its peculiarities was the straight line on the inside, with the curve upon the outside; that another was the *spring*, or curve on the bottom; another, the additional thickness over the place of the great toe; another, the level bottom side-wise, from the

9

shank, through the middle, forward ; another, the placing of the instep nearer to the side than is done in lasts of the present time. This was offered as a positively sure preventive of all those troubles arising from distortion of the toes, while also having a tendency to encourage feet already deformed in a return to their natural state.

From several of the positions thus taken, it necessarily follows that straight lasts are entirely wrong in formation and use, *and that nothing inferior to, or essentially different from, a right and left last of the form described, can fully serve the natural requirements of the foot.*

For flat-footedness the long heel was recommended as one great help toward recovering the natural position of the arch. A *long* heel is the next best thing to no heel at all. It supports the arch the most nearly as it is supported when the bare foot is pressed upon the ground or floor. Where this will not restore the shape, it will at least be likely to prevent the fault from becoming any worse. The other remedies—the proper exercise and full development of the muscles at the bottom of the foot, and the righting of it up when it treads inward—must be considered as in no way inferior, if not *superior*, to the first. Taken together, they offer a strong encouragement to those who wish to overcome the weakness, while they furnish a sure prevention of it where it does not already exist.

The importance of having lasts made expressly to fit

individual feet has not been sufficiently urged. Though many persons can get their feet very well fitted at any time without them, and others may be so situated that they can buy a handsomer and better article than they can get made, yet where a good shoemaker can be relied upon to make such a covering as is wanted, there is advantage in knowing how a good fit can always be obtained. This is by having a pair of lasts made as nearly right as possible, then allowing the shoemaker to test and correct them after making a first pair of boots or shoes on them, when they will be right for the remainder of a lifetime. The shoemaker may also, after making the first pair, have a pattern for any particular form of the upper, likewise corrected and made reliable for further use. The expense of such lasts is not great, and the custom shoemaker can himself furnish those from his own stock for a large proportion of his customers, altering and fitting them up as may be necessary, and supplying their places with others from the lastmaker. They will need to be so fitted up that they can be slightly raised or lessened in size for thick or thin stockings, or an increase or decrease of flesh. If a perfect fit is not made when they are used the second time, a further slight correction will insure it. After this there will be no dissatisfaction on the part of the buyer; no fear of loss by misfits on the part of the maker. Those who have any peculiar notion about their foot-apparel can be suited. There will be very little trouble from delay, or from getting the foot accustomed to

the boot when first worn. Still further, and better, the
danger of making corns, bunions, grown-in nails, and sore
insteps is reduced to almost nothing; for the covering,
being a good fit, is neither tight nor loose, and does not
pinch, cramp, or chafe any part of the foot.

All these considerations are much more forcible when
the feet differ from an ordinary size and shape. A ready-
made article to fit cannot be bought. It is often difficult
for even the best mechanic to make work that will fit
easily and handsomely upon feet that are flat, and have
corns and large joints besides—a combination of difficulties he is frequently called upon to meet. There is the
additional fact that many feet can seldom or never be
measured twice alike, for all feet vary in size under different conditions, and some of them a great deal; and
hence the uncertainty of being fitted by a shoemaker the
first time he is employed.* But when a last of the right

* To those custom shoemakers who continue trying to fit everybody
without any specially-made lasts it is suggested that in some of the
most difficult they make a *trial* shoe, the upper for it being cut from
some cheap material, such as cotton drilling for representing serge or
cloth, and split-leather or sheepskin for leather,uppers, while a piece
of insole-leather will answer for the bottom. The upper can be sewed
together without lining, only some eyelets being necessary for lacing,
and when drawn over such a last as is judged likely to fit the foot it
may be roughly fastened down all around with a waxed thread. After
trial on the customer's foot, the upper can be ripped off and the sole-
leather used for an insole or something else, while if the shoe fits badly
the last is easily modified, before making a permanent article. The
same plan might be tried with any new last designed for a particular
foot.

size, length, width, and general shape has been obtained, with all the corns, joints, sore insteps and other peculiarities fairly represented upon it, the owner may expect more comfort for the feet, and a better-looking boot, than has ever been realized for them before. But such a last cannot be made perfectly correct at first, and the customer must not be discouraged at finding a little difficulty. The final satisfaction will repay all the trouble.

A pair of lasts for *boots*, if made in the right way, with a good width at the shank (or just above it), while rather narrow at the top, and with a full amount of spring at the toe, can be used for making *shoes* and *slippers*, in ordinary cases, by filling up the shank with a piece of sole-leather in a way well known to custom shoemakers ; although the most perfect results are obtained by having a separate pair designed for slippers and low shoes. Those who have difficult feet had better limit themselves to one pair for all kinds of coverings.

There is hence no need of feet being badly fitted because they are badly shaped, if their possessors will act upon the suggestions given. Yet it must not be expected that big joints and flat insteps can be made *handsome* by any degree of skill ; they can be well fitted, but their shape remains visible.

A boot or shoe ought to fit easily, yet snugly and smoothly, all over the foot—around the heel and ankle as well as the forward part. There is no necessity for pinching the instep or crowding the toes ; no occasion for loose leather at the ankle and heel; no propriety in wrinkles over the instep of a flat foot, nor having a slipper loose at the sides. All *boots* must have wrinkles at the ankle, and all kinds of covering must have some across the foot at the joints. There need not be any of marked size elsewhere, nor should these be as large as they commonly are. A new boot should be put on with care to avoid making them.

The ease and grace of movement connected with feet in their normal condition, and when properly dressed, has been hinted at several times previously. This is a consideration almost entirely overlooked; yet it is not a thing of small importance. Everybody, in greater or less degree, admires grace and beauty. Nearly everyone who has a consciousness of being awkward in any way, suffers from that feeling or knowledge. This love of the beautiful is as much a part of human nature as conscience; and contributes as much to our pleasure as almost any other sentiment or affection. When turned more in this direction, as it should be, it will appreciate beauty in the feet as quickly as elsewhere. Its influence must be brought to bear in developing the true and elegant in this department, no less than in others. It should appreciate a well-formed foot, whether small or large; and a graceful, easy step in the street as well as in the ball-room. Let the shuffling or stamping gait of flat-footed persons generally, be contrasted with the light yet dignified carriage of those whose feet are properly arched; let the stiff walk of a man in tight boots be noticed, and then the step of one who goes along in a pair of light, easy shoes with low heels. The difference in each of these cases will be very plain. A person cannot walk easily and handsomely—much less *run*—in boots that are uncomfortable, or with corns and sore joints crying out at every step. High heels necessarily give an unnatural character to the step, because the heel of the foot does not come near the surface, as Nature intended. The weight of the body is thrown too much upon the forward part of the foot, which would seem likely to have some tendency toward breaking it down, *while it prevents that very spring upon the ball and toes which is the most essential thing in graceful walking.**

* The effects upon the foot are not the only bad results springing from heels that are extremely high. The work of Dr. C. F. Taylor has already been quoted from to show the influence of weak ankles in developing lateral curvature of the spine. We also find in it some hints concerning *stoop-shoulders*, which are thus expressed.

" Man has a much narrower base of sustentation than most other animals, which renders it important that that base should not be lessened by cramping the feet in narrow shoes, rendering progression difficult, awkward, and quickly fatiguing. But probably the most serious fault in the feet-coverings is the elevated heel often given to them. By elevating the heel, besides the still narrower base given, whether in progression or standing, the anatomical relations of the whole body as an instrument of locomotion are materially changed. As in lateral curvature of the spine, a deviation from the proper position at one point may cause several other compensating curves at other points, so an improper position of one part of the locomotive apparatus will cause a succession of other false positions of other parts. By elevating the heel and constantly keeping the flexors of the feet [the muscles on the upper side] on the stretch, relief to them is instinctively sought by a slight flexion at the knee; this would

Besides this, it is known that high heels *prevent the full growth of the calf of the leg,* by preventing the full exercise of those muscles which raise the heel at every step. As it is kept constantly raised already by an inch and a half of leather under it, of course there is less required of the muscles, and they are decreased in size.

Stiffness, also, has a decided effect upon the carriage of the body. One who has always worn stiff, clumsy footgear has a stiff, awkward walk, because all the muscles of the foot and leg brought into play by natural walking have been interfered with and cramped by the miserable clogs on the feet. As these will bend, or allow the foot to bend, but very little, there can be but little use of the muscles which form the calf of the leg and raise the heel. Hence

destroy the perpendicularity of the figure, were not another slight flexion made at the hips ; but as this would throw the trunk forward, still another flexion backward is required, and then forward, etc. But in the spinal column a compromise is effected by a forward curve and inclination of the head. Thus, high heels tend to produce and permanently establish a succession of zigzags from the ankles upward, with the weight of the body supported by the tension of the muscles, and not, as in erect stature, by the bony framework."— *Theory and Practice of the Movement-Cure,* p. 75.

The position here described is an approach to that assumed by old people—those " bent over by age "—who are unable from weakness to stand upright. The abdominal muscles are relaxed, the chest sinks, the head falls forward, and the spine adapts itself by bending at the neck and shoulders. The author goes on to show that these effects are felt more sensibly by women than by men, and that their diseases and weaknesses are thus rendered more aggravated, and the complete cure of them retarded or prevented by the wearing of high heels.

the calf remains weak and undeveloped, instead of pre-
senting the full, round, muscular appearance it shows in a
well-developed leg, and which is so necessary to a light,
easy, elastic step, and graceful movement.

The fashionable world—those people whom the earnest
thinker and the practical utilitarian look upon almost as
useless idlers in the community—still have their superiority in one direction, over the thinker or business man,
which must be fairly acknowledged. They are artists in
the matter of dress and personal ornamentation. They
possess that taste and keen sense of the beautiful which
forms everything around them into elegance, grace, and
charm. Though they sometimes sacrifice strength and
usefulness, and often go to foolish extremes, as do the
plainer sort in an opposite way, yet they generally manifest
a propriety in dress and surroundings which compels the
admiration even of those sensible and steady ones who
think so highly of the useful, but depreciate the value of
beauty.

To the fashionable class, then, no less than to others
we appeal to adopt a fashion in dressing the feet which
will tend strongly to develop beauty in their *form and
appearance*, and grace in all their *movements*. What this
is, has been sufficiently well explained. It may be added
that no one should be satisfied without a good fit, and an
article as tasteful and carefully selected as anything that
is wo rn upon the head, or any other part of the person.
The foot has the same right to be well dressed that is
possessed by any other portion of the body.

A shape of the sole that would be a compromise between the common form and the correct one, has been suggested for the benefit of those who could not be persuaded to have anything better. This is a good one for such feet as are somewhat distorted at the toes, and whose owners are not disposed to attempt any correction. But we protest against putting anything less perfect than the "Excelsior" upon *young* feet, that are still undeformed, and hence entitled to a covering that will correspond. Parents have no right to treat their children in such a way as to induce any of the troubles that have been described. But this they are almost sure to do, in greater or less degree, by compelling them to wear the ordinary boot and shoe. It is true the better kind cannot be obtained ready-made at first, though the demand will produce them in a reasonable time, yet some approach to the true thing can be made by a shoemaker of intelligence and ingenuity, even though, in the absence of proper lasts, he is obliged to alter and improve some which he already has. Some day the better article will be both obtainable and inexpensive. In the mean time those most interested must take the best substitute within their reach—that which comes nearest the true standard.

CHAPTER X.

Miscellaneous—Criticism of Different Forms and Fashions—Elasticity—Sensitiveness—Rubbers and Waterproof Leather—Cure for
Sweating—Qualities of a good Covering.

IT has been said that fashion should never be allowed
to change the shape of the sole, or interfere with the
form of the lasts used in the construction of the foot's
coverings. This restriction, however, does not apply to
the materials of which they are made, nor the form into
which the *uppers* may be cut. The latter may be of a great
variety of forms, and the material of almost any kind or
quality, and of all colours and descriptions of ornamentation. Yet there are many particulars that are matters of
style now, which will give way to something different in
another year, or in two or three years. Each of the different
kinds of boots has certain peculiar advantages which, in
addition to its being fashionable, contribute to make it
popular. The side-spring boot, that has been a favourite
so long, seldom slips at the heel, and this is a decidedly
good point ; it also, by fitting closely at the ankles, gives
a feeling of snugness and security which is comfortable,

while it admits of perfect freedom in all movements of the ankle in walking. There is less trouble in putting it on and off than with most other descriptions of boots and shoes which is a recommendation to many people who value time or dislike extra labour.

The *Balmoral boot* for ladies has its recommendation in its *superiority of fit.* This has made, and keeps it, a favourite, causing it to be more generally worn than any other. The manner of lacing enables the wearer to draw it smooth and snug over the instep and around the heel and ankle— an advantage possessed by no other, except, partially, by the side-laced boot ; which is likely to come again into favour,

The *Polish boot* takes the place of the Balmoral when a greater height upon the leg is required. There is no other difference in its form, and the quality of fit is the same. Its worst disadvantage is the amount of time required in lacing and unlacing it, although, when made of thick leather, it may have a slight cramping effect upon the muscles of the ankle.

The *Button boot,* often called the Hungarian, when cut high like the Polish, is at this time the most fashionable. It is quite as handsome, but has not usually the neatness of fit which the Balmoral possesses.

One style, not generally introduced, but of which a pair has been made occasionally, is superior to the Polish or Hungarian in that there is only half as much trouble in lacing. It may be made very high—thirteen inches, if desired—being laced or buttoned about as far up as the Balmoral, when the upper part of one quarter is folded over past the opening, and fastened with two or three handsome clasps attached to elastic straps, which give and retract sufficiently to accommodate the action of the leg, while at the same time the leg is snugly fitted. This is a good heavy winter boot for ladies, where an extreme height or length of leg is in demand. The *Highland buckle* is similar to it, the part that laps over being fastened with one inelastic strap. We have also noticed a high boot made with gores like the side-spring—one at the ankle and two above on each side—which would seem to be a very convenient thing to put on, but one that needs the best gores to make it serviceable. It is not probable that either of these varieties will be extensively popular. The first is of the three the most deserving.

The quality needed by all laced, buckled, or buttoned boots is *elasticity* at the leg, ankle, or instep, such as is possessed at one point—the ankle—by the side-spring. A great advantage would be gained if this elasticity could be extended down even to the ball or joint. One purpose of it is *to give free play to the muscles of the leg and ankle, and also allow the foot to lengthen and spread without hindrance as its arches expand under the weight of the body in walking or standing; and another is to keep the upper closely drawn over all parts of the foot, ankle, and leg, when the arches are contracted and the muscles inactive, as in a state of rest; both objects—ease to the foot and*

beauty of fit—being secured by the same means. Buckle
and button boots for gentlemen, with this quality supplied at the ankle by a narrow goring on one side of it,
while the buckles or buttons are on the other side, have
lately been made. The gored Oxford shoe supplies the
elasticity at the instep. Perhaps some other style can be
invented that will do as much for the ball and transverse
arch as these kinds have done for the parts above. Any
boot or shoe with this peculiarity is superior to the same
thing without it. It must not, of course, be supposed
that such a shoe will fit a thick or a slim foot equally well,
for the elastic may be too tight for ease in one case, and too
loose for a good fit in the other.

In connection with this matter, strong elastic cords for
laces are suggested as worthy of a trial in Balmoral and
Polish boots. If successful, they accomplish the same
result as elastic goring, and, besides, may be drawn
tightly or loosely to meet the defect of the boot, or suit
the convenience or taste of the wearer.

Cloth and leather materials are joined together in
ladies' work in all sorts of proportions. In regard to this
practice it may be said that those kinds of shoes in which
the higher part is made of cloth or lasting, and the lower
and forward parts of leather, are to be preferred for one
reason : the softer part at the ankle allows of more freedom and ease to the muscles, while the leather below
serves all the purposes it would if extending throughout,
and thus the advantages of both are combined. There is

no difficulty in making this union, whatever the *cut* of the boot may be—whether gored, laced, or buttoned.

Tender feet may find what suits their wants in the softer kinds of kid and morocco, when cloth is not preferred. There is no reason why a woman's boot, though a heavy one, should be hard and stiff; as a good quality of oiled morocco, pebbled calf, or calf-kid leather, to be obtained almost anywhere, will commonly be found pliable enough, even for moderately sensitive corns. Still more softness may be given by double linings of flannel.

There is no leather worn by ladies that is water-proof, and that quality ought not to be expected. Their heaviest boots are made with a double sole and double upper, which give additional warmth, and protect against ordinary dampness. But the only thing they have as a sure protection against wet is rubber. Rubber sandals or shoes for the sidewalk or a rainy day, and high rubber boots for snow, are a complete security.

Men are, in this respect, better provided for. There are several kinds of leather worn by them which, if saturated with grease or special preparations, will be water-proof, though exposed for a considerable time. They have the benefit of rubber besides.

The Napoleon tongued boot, for a heavy one, is supposed to have a superiority of fit about the ankle, and is more tasteful in a general way.

The double-footed boot is considered, with some reason, to be *warmer* than a single one of the same thickness.

For men's feet that are very sensitive to cold, perhaps the best thing is a doubled boot, having the inside part, or foot-lining, made of fur-calf—calf skin dressed with the hair on—or some other kind of fur. Arctic overshoes are very excellent for riding in cold weather, provided they are not too small. Cork soles, covered with wool or flannel, for either sex, are another help toward keeping the feet warm, with which, in addition to flannel linings and other provisions, the most cold-footed ought to be tolerably comfortable. It must not, however, be expected to keep the feet warm in any kind of a covering that is *tight.*

But as this kind of sensitiveness is, in healthy persons, very much a matter of habit, it is perhaps quite as well for such to accustom themselves to wearing an ordinary doubled boot through the winter, unless much exposed, and put on a light boot, shoe, or gaiter for the summer. Appropriateness and adaptation to weather or circumstances are always to be considered. A heavy leather boot with double sole is as much out of place and time in a warm day, as a light cloth gaiter in a snow-storm. While the latter would expose the foot unnecessarily, the first, besides being uncomfortable, keeps the foot in an unnaturally sensitive condition. It is not intended to make any suggestions to *invalids.* We only state the well-known rule that exposure to cold makes the feet, or any other part of the body, more hardy, when there is an ordinary state of health, or sufficient blood in the system to be easily drawn to the surface by this demand. Where there is too little vitality for this, the experience of the person or the counsel of the physician is the best guide. So also in regard to dampness or wetting the feet. While making no law for sickly or feeble constitutions, it seems to us very evident that the more often the feet are exposed to damp or wet, the greater the ability acquired by the system to resist it ;* and that when the feet happen to get wet only occasionally, the consequences of the exposure are proportionately more serious. It is probable that if care were taken to keep the feet *comfortably warm* when wet, either by exercise, as in walking, or in some other manner, there would be very little danger from the wet alone, unless in cases of invalid feebleness, or where they were dampened so seldom that the intelligence of the physical system was unprepared for such an occurrence.

One of the well-established facts of physiology is that anything worn upon the feet which, like rubber or patent leather, prevents the passing off of the insensible perspiration,

* It may become an important problem to the physiologist and physician to determine whether the same law does not hold good in respect to *whatever* is naturally injurious to the human constitution *in any way*, so long as its resisting power *is not overbalanced*. If all kinds of unhealthy conditions, surroundings, and exposures can be made to produce the good effects of healthful stimulation when made use of to the proper extent, however little that may be, while only past that limit they become destructive, then a change will come over a great many notions and practices. Some facts are reconciled by such a theory which are otherwise quite contradictory.

10

is detrimental to the health. Those who regard the organic laws as having any sacredness, will not use patent leather boots covering the whole foot, for constant wear, but limit them to particular occasions. Rubbers ought to be removed, and something else substituted in their place, as soon as the feet come out of the wet which occasions their being put on. The same is true of all boots that are waterproof. They should be worn only when times of exposure make them necessary. This is sufficiently well known with regard to rubbers; but few know that leather boots are objectionable, for the same reason, in proportion as they are watertight. There are comparatively few of them which are perfectly so; yet there are many, which, worn as they are, day after day, in dry weather as well as wet, must, by retaining a large part of the foot's perspiration, have an unhealthful effect. It is a good practice to bathe the feet after removing a pair of waterproof boots which have been worn during the day. With many men this is a necessity, and it would be such with many more if they knew all the requirements of the laws of hygiene, to say nothing of any other reason. To give the boots themselves a washing-out occasionally might be advantageous. The feet must be allowed to perspire naturally, or the skin in some other part is liable to be overtasked; and it is stated by medical authorities that skin diseases have been produced by neglect of the feet in this particular.

The following cure for abnormal sweating of the feet is taken from one of our first-class periodicals;* and from the

* *Appleton's Journal*—department devoted to Science.

nature of the remedy it would seem that it ought to have the effect indicated.

" Pulverized tannin sprinkled inside the boots or shoes in three days prevents tender feet from perspiring and blistering. Tanning thus applied, rapidly strengthens and hardens the skin, softened by the simultaneous action of moisture and heat ; perspiration being thus reduced to the proper degree, without its healthy action being in the slightest interfered with, the exhalations as a matter of course cease to be offensive. The cessation of disagreeable odours is explained by the fact that the products of the ammoniacal decomposition of the skin are immediately combined with the tannin and so carried off."

Rubber-soled shoes for ladies, with leather or other material for the uppers, have been manufactured to a slight extent ; and, as far as we know, are a success. The objection on account of health does not apply to them seriously, because the rubber is at the bottom. Possibly, however, an uncomfortable effect may be produced upon the sole of the foot.

Water-proof serge or lasting, also, is among the late inventions. It is claimed to be sufficiently porous to allow the escape of perspiration, yet water-proof under all ordinary exposure. The two qualities are incompatible and if really water-proof it is only fit, like rubber, to be worn occasionally.

Cloth materials of different kinds have been much worn. They permit a partial saving of leather, and are equally handsome. They are light, soft, may be made sufficiently warm, and are far more favourable to health. They answer nearly every requirement for a good shoe, except the defence against dampness; and their wearing ought to be encouraged. The defect named must be supplied by rubbers.

Nearly all the coarser and cheaper kinds of men's shoe goods have the bad quality of general stiffness. Their wearing makes, in a very decided and proper sense, *stiff feet.* They are all the worse for having pegged soles. Whether the soles are curved or straight makes not much difference, for the stiffness prevents the use of either the upper or lower set of the foot's muscles. As these goods can not be generally manufactured at the present time without being made stiff by pegs, in addition to the firmness of the leather, there is but little chance for improvement. Those obliged to wear them are advised to do so only so far as they are compelled, and to keep the upper parts in as pliable a condition as possible by frequent applications of oil. It is to be hoped that something softer will some time take their place.

The value of all these various styles, and of any other that may come up hereafter, may be tested by the presence or absence of the following general qualities: sufficient porosity of the upper to admit the passage of the insensible perspiration; softness and pliability sufficient to allow of ease and comfort to the foot in all its movements; flexibility and elasticity that will yield to accommodate the action of the muscles at the ankle and top of the foot, yet draw the upper tight enough to fit smoothly; general good shape and proportion ; flexibility of sole ; strength for protection and service. The more of these there can be combined into any species of foot-clothing the better will the foot be protected and preserved, and at the least expense of money and trouble in proportion to the benefit gained.

THE END.

www.ingramcontent.com/pod-product-compliance
Lightning Source LLC
Chambersburg PA
CBHW031434270326
41930CB00007B/705